ATKINS DIET 2025

110 Quick Recipes Discover the Nutritional Trends of the Future a Complete Guide to Weight Loss Long-Lasting Wellbeing an Active Life

KLARLOCK

DISCLAIMER

This book aims to provide useful and informative material on the topics covered in the publication. It is sold with the understanding that the author and publisher are not engaged in rendering any personal medical, health care, or other professional services in the book. The reader should consult his or her physician, health care provider, or other competent professional before adopting any suggestions in this book or drawing any conclusions. The author and publisher expressly disclaim any responsibility for any liability, loss, or risk, personal or otherwise, arising, directly or indirectly, from the use and application of any contents of this book.

NOTE

All the recipes in this book are designed for four people. For this quantity, the ingredients indicated in the recipes must be considered. If you need to change the portion, it is recommended to proportionally adjust the doses of the ingredients. It is also recommended to carefully follow the preparation and cooking instructions to obtain the best result. In the context of this book, when we refer to "a cup" as a unit of measurement for ingredients, we mean using a standard kitchen cup with a capacity of approximately 240 milliliters. It is essential to use a measuring cup to get the right quantities of ingredients. If you don't have a measuring cup, you can use a graduated measuring cup, making sure to correctly correspond to the proportions indicated. Here are some examples 1 Cup of flour 100 gr. 1 cup of rice 200 gr. 1 Cup of Quinoa 200 gr

TABLE OF CONTENT

MAINTAIN LONG-TERM SUCCESS

RECIPES APPETIZERS

67 GRILLED CHICKEN SALAD WITH
MAYONNAISE

69 SMOKED SALMON CANAPES WITH
CREAM CHEESE

71 RAW HAM WITH MELON

73 GRILLED CHICKEN SKEWERS WITH
PEPPERS

75 LIVER PATÉ WITH CELERY CROUTTONS

77 OLIVES STUFFED WITH CHEESE

78 CANNED MACKEREL WITH AVOCADO
AND LIME

80 STUFFED COURGETTES WITH MINCED
MEAT

82 BROCCOLI AND CHEESE FLAN

84 ROASTED PEPPER ROLLS WITH RICOTTA

86 OCTOPUS SALAD WITH CELERY AND
LEMON

88 ASPARAGUS WRAPPED IN HAM

90 SALMON MOUSSE WITH DRIED
TOMATOES

RECIPES FIRST DISHES

186 MUSHROOM SOUP WITH CREAM AND PARSLEY

188 CHICKEN SALAD WITH GRILLED VEGETABLES AND FETA CHEESE

190 ZUCCHINI LINGUINE WITH TOMATO SAUCE AND OVEN COOKED CHICKEN

192 TOMATO SOUP WITH SHRIMP AND BASIL

194 TUNA SALAD WITH BOILED EGGS AND AVOCADO

196 CUCUMBER TAGLIOLINI WITH TUNA SAUCE AND DRIED TOMATOES

198 CAULIFLOWER RICE WITH GRILLED CHICKEN AND SPINACH

200 VEGETABLE SOUP WITH TURKEY MEATBALLS WITH LEMON

202 COURGETTE PAD THAI WITH CHICKEN AND PEANUT SAUCE

205 CHICKEN SALAD WITH AVOCADO, DRIED TOMATOES AND FETA CHEESE

207 CAULIFLOWER RISOTTO WITH CRISPY BACON AND GRATED CHEESE

210 TOMATO SOUP WITH SHRIMP AND BASIL

212 TUNA SALAD WITH AVOCADO, CUCUMBERS AND BLACK OLIVES

214 CUCUMBER NOODLES WITH TOMATO SAUCE AND BAKED SAUSAGE

RECIPES SECOND DISHES

217 GRILLED CHICKEN WITH AVOCADO SAUCE

219 GRILLED BEEF STEAK WITH GRILLED VEGETABLES

221 LEMON CHICKEN BREAST WITH SAUTEED SPINACH

223 GRILLED SALMON WITH AVOCADO SAUCE

225 BAKED TURKEY MEATBALLS WITH MIXED SALAD

227 PORK CHOPS WITH MUSHROOM SAUCE AND STEAMED BROCCOLI

230 ROAST CHICKEN WITH ARUGULA AND TOMATO SALAD

232 SOLE IN PIECE WITH STEAMED VEGETABLES

234 GRILLED PRAWN SKEWERS WITH SAUTEED COURGETTES

236 PORK FILLET WITH MUSTARD SAUCE AND BAKED CAULIFLOWER

238 CHICKEN CACCIATORA WITH ROASTED PEPPERS

241 GRILLED TUNA WITH LIME SAUCE AND CUCUMBER SALAD

243 LAMB CHOPS WITH GRILLED ASPARAGUS

245 CURRY CHICKEN WITH BAKED CAULIFLOWER

247 BAKED SALMON WITH AVOCADO SAUCE AND SPINACH SALAD

249 BAKED BEEF MEATBALLS WITH GRATINUM COURGETTES

252 BAKED COD WITH TOMATO SAUCE AND ARUGULA SALAD

SIDE DISH RECIPES

INTRODUCTION TO THE ATKINS DIET

Weight Loss Fundamentals and Goals

The Atkins Diet: A low-carb, high-protein, high-fat diet designed to put the body into a metabolic state called ketosis. In this state, the body burns fat as its primary source of energy, instead of glucose derived from carbohydrates, leading to rapid weight loss.

Fundamental principles:

Drastic reduction in carbohydrates: Limit carbohydrate intake to 20-50 grams per day, depending on the phase of the diet. Increase protein intake: Consume lean protein from meat, poultry, fish, eggs and dairy products to maintain muscle mass and satiety. Healthy fats as a primary source of energy:

Include healthy fats like olive oil, avocado, nuts and seeds in your diet to promote satiety and overall health.

Weight loss goals:

Rapid initial weight loss: Ketosis can lead to rapid weight loss, especially of water and glycogen stored in the liver and muscles. Steady weight loss: As your body adapts to ketosis, weight loss may slow down, but it should still occur consistently over time. Improved metabolic health: The Atkins diet can improve risk factors for heart disease, such as cholesterol and blood pressure, and reduce blood sugar levels.

The Atkins diet can be an effective way to lose weight and improve health for some people. However, it's important to talk to your doctor before starting any new diet, especially if you have pre-existing medical conditions. It is essential to follow your diet correctly to avoid potential health risks. In the next chapters, we'll delve deeper into the Atkins diet and give you the information you need to make an informed decision about whether it's right for you.

WHAT IS THE ATKINS DIET

The Atkins diet is a dietary approach based on reducing carbohydrates and increasing the intake of proteins and healthy fats. It was developed by Dr. Robert C. Atkins in the 1970s and has proven popular for weight loss and appetite control. The Atkins diet is based on the theory that excessive intake of carbohydrates, especially those with a high glycemic index, can cause blood sugar spikes and promote the formation of fat deposits. By reducing your carbohydrate intake, you aim to keep your blood sugar levels stable and encourage your body to use fat stores as an energy source. In the initial phase, called the induction phase, you strictly limit your carbohydrate intake to less than 20 grams per day. During this phase, the body enters a state of ketosis, in which it primarily burns fat for energy.

Next, gradually add healthy carbohydrates, such as low-carb vegetables, berries, and low-fat dairy products. The Atkins diet emphasizes eating high-quality proteins, such as lean meats, fish, eggs and dairy products. Additionally, encourage the use of healthy fats, such as olive oil, avocado, nuts and seeds. The goal is to create balanced, satiating meals that help control appetite and keep blood sugar levels stable. One of the key points of the Atkins diet is the elimination of refined sugars and white flour, as well as processed and packaged foods that contain added carbohydrates. We encourage you to choose whole, fresh, unprocessed foods for maximum nutritional benefit.

Many people follow the Atkins diet to lose weight, but it is claimed to offer other benefits as well, such as lowering blood sugar levels, improving triglyceride and "good" cholesterol (HDL) levels, and stabilizing energy throughout the day . In conclusion, the Atkins diet is a dietary approach based on reducing carbohydrates and increasing the intake of proteins and healthy fats. It was developed to help people lose weight, control appetite and stabilize blood sugar levels. However, it is crucial to consult a doctor before starting any significant diet program.

BENEFITS OF THE ATKINS DIET

The Atkins diet is touted to offer several health and wellness benefits, particularly weight loss. Let's look at some of the potential benefits you may experience:

1. Rapid initial weight loss:

One of the hallmarks of the Atkins diet is its ability to induce rapid weight loss, especially at first. This is because drastically restricting carbohydrates causes the body to enter ketosis, a state in which it begins burning stored fat for energy instead of glucose derived from carbohydrates. This process can lead to significant initial weight loss, often consisting of water and glycogen stored in the liver and muscles.

2. Improved blood sugar:

The Atkins diet may be beneficial for people with blood sugar problems, such as predibetes or type 2 diabetes. By reducing the intake of carbohydrates, which are broken down into glucose in the blood, the Atkins diet can help keep levels in check of blood sugar.

3. Greater sense of satiety:

The Atkins diet emphasizes protein and healthy fats, which are nutrients known to promote satiety and reduce hunger. This can lead to lower overall calorie consumption and more sustainable weight loss over time.

4. Reduced Appetite and Cravings for Sugary Foods:

By limiting refined carbohydrates and added sugars, the Atkins diet can help reduce cravings for sugary and starchy foods. This can be helpful for those who struggle with emotional hunger or cravings for specific foods. It's important to keep in mind that research on the Atkins diet is mixed. While it may offer some short-term benefits, there are also potential drawbacks to consider before starting this diet.

PHASES OF THE ATKINS DIET

Understand the process of induction, weight loss, balance and maintenance.

The Atkins diet is a low-carbohydrate diet, created by Dr. Robert C. Atkins in the 1970s, that focuses on protein and healthy fats for weight loss. It is based on the principle of causing the body to enter a metabolic state called ketosis.

The Atkins diet is structured into four progressive phases:

1. Induction (2 weeks) : Extremely low carbohydrate consumption, less than 20 grams per day. This initial period aims to rapidly induce ketosis.

The induction phase of the Atkins Diet

2. Weight Loss : Gradually increase carbohydrate intake to 25-50 grams per day while continuing to lose weight.

Opens in a new window

3. Pre-maintenance : Further increase carbohydrate intake to 50-100 grams per day. In this phase, vegetables rich in carbohydrates and some types of fruit are gradually introduced.

The premaintenance phase of the Atkins Diet

4. Maintenance : Increasing carbohydrate intake to a personalized maintenance level, which allows you to maintain the weight achieved. The goal is to find the lowest level of net carbs that still allows you to lose or maintain weight.

FOODS ALLOWED AND RESTRICTED ON THE ATKINS DIET

A Detailed Guide

The Atkins diet is a low-carb diet that aims to get the body to burn fat as its primary energy source, rather than carbohydrates. It is based on the principle of ketosis, a metabolic state in which the liver produces ketones from fats for the body's energy needs. The Atkins diet is divided into four phases: Induction, Weight Loss, Pre-Maintenance and Maintenance. Each phase has a specific daily carbohydrate limit and a list of allowed and restricted foods.

Allowed foods: In all phases:

Meat: Beef, pork, chicken, turkey, lamb, game, fish and seafood Eggs: Whole eggs, any way cooked

Healthy Fats: Olive oil, avocado oil, butter, cream, nuts and seeds

Low-carb vegetables: Leafy greens (spinach, lettuce, kale), broccoli, cauliflower, zucchini, cucumbers, peppers

Low-carb fruits: Berries (strawberries, raspberries, blueberries), avocados, grapefruits

Cheeses: Whole cheeses (cheddar, mozzarella, parmesan)

Full-fat yogurt: Full-fat Greek yogurt, sugar-free yogurt

Restricted Foods: In all stages:

Cereals: Bread, pasta, rice, cereals, oats

Sugars and sweets: Candy, cookies, cakes, ice cream, table sugar, maple syrup, honey
Fruits high in sugar: Bananas, grapes, mango, oranges, pineapple

Sweetened drinks: Fruit juices, carbonated drinks, energy drinks, sweetened tea, sweetened coffee

Processed foods: French fries, packaged snacks, fast food

In the early stages (Induction and Weight Loss):

High-Carbohydrate Vegetables: Potatoes, sweet potatoes, beets, carrots, corn

Legumes: Beans, lentils, chickpeas

Additionally, it's important to remember that the Atkins diet isn't right for everyone. Some people, such as pregnant or breastfeeding women, people with certain medical conditions, or individuals with eating disorders, should avoid this diet.

INDUCTION TO THE ATKINS DIET

The induction phase of the Atkins diet is the most restrictive and is the initial one, designed to last about two weeks. During this time, the goal is to push your body into ketosis by drastically limiting your carbohydrate intake.

Carb Limit:

Less than 20 grams of net carbohydrates per day: It is important to specify "net" because only digestible carbohydrates are considered, subtracting dietary fiber from the total carbohydrates. Fiber is not fully absorbed by the body and therefore does not contribute significantly to calorie intake.

Allowed foods:

Protein: Fatty meats (beef, pork, lamb), poultry (chicken, turkey), fatty fish (salmon, tuna), whole eggs

Healthy Fats: Olive oil, avocado oil, butter, cream, nuts and oil seeds

Low-carb vegetables: Leafy greens (spinach, kale), broccoli, cauliflower, zucchini, asparagus, celery

Water and calorie-free drinks: Black coffee or unsweetened tea

Foods to avoid:

Cereals: Bread, pasta, rice, breakfast cereals, oats

Sugars and sweets: Candy, biscuits, cakes, ice cream, table sugar, maple syrup, honey

Fruit: Most fruits are too high in sugar for this phase.

High-Carbohydrate Vegetables: Potatoes, sweet potatoes, beets, carrots, corn

Legumes: Beans, lentils, chickpeas

Sugary drinks: Fruit juices, soft drinks

sodas, energy drinks, sweetened tea, sweetened coffee Starchy foods: French fries, packaged snacks, fast food

Tips for the induction phase:

Drink plenty of water: Water is crucial for overall health and helps flush out excess ketones produced during ketosis. Supplement electrolytes: Carbohydrate restriction can lead to a loss of electrolytes such as sodium, potassium and magnesium. You may need to supplement these minerals with supplements or foods rich in them. Plan your meals: Planning your meals and snacks in advance will help you resist temptation and stay on track with your diet. It is important to remember that the induction phase is only the first part of the Atkins diet. After the initial two weeks, you move into the weight loss phase where your carbohydrate intake is gradually increased to aid in weight loss while still causing your body to burn fat.

CARBOHYDRATE MANAGEMENT

Strategies for monitoring carbohydrate intake and maximizing weight loss. Carbohydrate management is a fundamental aspect of the Atkins diet, as it allows you to induce and maintain ketosis, the metabolic state that favors the burning of fat as a primary energy source.

The phases of the Atkins diet and the carbohydrate limit: The Atkins diet is divided into four phases, each with a specific daily net carbohydrate limit:

Induction: Less than 20 grams of net carbs per day (about 2 weeks)

Weight Loss: Gradually increase net carbs by 5 grams per week until you reach your "critical carb level for weight loss" (the point at which you stop losing weight)

Pre-Maintenance: Gradually increase net carbs by 10 grams per week until weight loss stabilizes

Maintenance: Intake of net carbohydrates that maintain ketosis and desired body weight

Net Carbs Calculation:

To determine your net carbs, you need to subtract dietary fiber from your total carbs. Fiber is not fully absorbed by the body and therefore does not contribute significantly to calorie intake.

Example:

If a food has 15 grams of total carbohydrates and 5 grams of fiber, the net carbohydrates would be:

15 grams total carbs - 5 grams fiber = 10 grams net carbs

Choosing the right carbohydrates: Not all carbohydrates are created equal on the Atkins diet. It is important to choose foods rich in fiber and nutrients and limit those with a high content of sugars and refined starches.

Examples of allowed carbohydrate foods:

Low-carb vegetables: Leafy greens, broccoli, cauliflower, zucchini, peppers

Low sugar fruits: Berries, avocados, grapefruits

Healthy Fats: Olive oil, avocado oil, butter, cream, nuts and seeds

Proteins: Meat, fish, eggs

Examples of carbohydrate foods to limit:

Cereals: Bread, pasta, rice, breakfast cereals

Sugars and sweets: Candy, biscuits, cakes, ice cream, table sugar, maple syrup, honey

Fruits high in sugar: Bananas, grapes, mango, oranges, pineapple

High-Carbohydrate Vegetables: Potatoes, sweet potatoes, beets, carrots, corn

Legumes: Beans, lentils, chickpeas

Carb Management Tips:

Read food labels carefully: Pay attention to the net carbohydrate content and dietary fiber on each food. Plan your meals: Planning your meals and snacks in advance helps you make informed choices and stay within your carbohydrate limits. Use a food measuring cup: Use a measuring cup to properly portion foods and control your carbohydrate intake. Listen to your body: Pay attention to how you feel and adjust your carbohydrate intake if necessary.

IMPROVE RESULTS WITH EXERCISE

How to integrate a fitness program into the Atkins diet to maximize results, Improve Results with Exercise in the Atkins Diet Exercise is an important complement to the Atkins diet for optimal results in terms of weight loss and improved health general.

Benefits of Exercise During the Atkins Diet:

Increased calorie burn: Physical activity burns excess calories, promoting weight loss and muscle definition.

Increased insulin sensitivity: Exercise helps improve insulin sensitivity, allowing the body to use carbohydrates more efficiently and keep blood sugar levels stable. Stress Reduction: Physical activity helps reduce stress, which can hinder weight loss and overall health. Improved muscle tone: Strength exercise helps build and maintain muscle mass, which in turn increases basal metabolic rate and promotes calorie burning even at rest. Increased energy: Exercise increases energy levels and reduces tiredness, which can be a common side effect of starting the Atkins diet.

Recommended types of exercise:

Strength Exercise: Training with weights or your own body helps build and maintain muscle mass, which is important for a healthy metabolism and body definition. Daily activities: Increasing daily physical activity, such as taking the stairs or walking instead of taking the elevator, can significantly help burn calories.

Tips for Exercise During the Atkins Diet:

Listen to your body: There is no need to overdo exercise, especially at the beginning of the Atkins diet. Start with moderate activities and gradually increase the intensity and duration of workouts over time.

Stay hydrated: Drinking plenty of water before, during and after exercise is key to preventing dehydration.

Eat properly: Make sure you consume enough calories and nutrients to support physical activity. It is important to include protein and healthy fats in your diet to aid muscle recovery.

Get enough rest: Rest is important to allow your body to recover from exercise and prepare for the next workout. Consult a doctor or personal trainer.

MAINTAINING LONG-TERM SUCCESS

Strategies for maintaining weight gain and living a healthy lifestyle for the long term. Maintaining long-term success with the Atkins Diet requires ongoing commitment and a holistic approach that goes

beyond simple carbohydrate restriction. Here are some key tips to help you maintain your results and live a healthy lifestyle: 1. Find your carbohydrate maintenance level:

Pre-Maintenance Phase: Gradually increase net carbs by 10 grams per week until weight loss stabilizes.

Maintenance Phase: Eat the amount of net carbs that maintains ketosis and your desired body weight.

Listen to your body: Monitor your weight, energy levels and ketosis to adjust your carbohydrate intake individually.

2. Make smart food choices:

Focus on whole, unprocessed foods: Choose meats, fish, eggs, low-carb vegetables, healthy fats and low-sugar fruits. Limit processed foods, added sugars, and refined flours: These foods can easily derail the ketosis process and lead to weight gain. Learning to cook: Cooking at home allows you to control the ingredients and quality of the food. Practice moderation: Occasionally enjoying indulgent foods in moderation can help maintain long-term motivation.

3. Maintain regular physical exercise: Find enjoyable physical activity: Choose activities that you enjoy to make them more sustainable over time.

**Combine cardio and strength exercises:
Cardio training burns calories and promotes
fat loss, while strength training helps build
and maintain muscle mass. Aim for at least
30 minutes of moderate intensity exercise
most days of the week: This can be broken
up into shorter sessions throughout the day.**

**4. Prioritize adequate sleep and stress
management:**

**Aim for 7-8 hours of quality sleep each night:
Sleep deprivation can alter hormones that
regulate appetite and metabolism. Practice
stress reduction techniques: Stress can lead
to emotional eating and hinder weight loss
efforts. Find healthy ways to manage stress,
such as yoga, meditation, or spending time in
nature.**

RECIPES APPETIZERS

COURGETTE CARPACCIO WITH GOAT'S CHEESE

45

Preparation time: 10 minutes

Cooking time: 0 minutes

(if you don't grill the courgettes)

Doses for: 4 people

Ingredients:

2 medium courgettes

60 ml olive oil

30 ml lemon juice

1 clove garlic, minced

Salt and pepper to taste

100g goat's cheese, crumbled

Fresh basil, for garnish

Preparation:

Thinly slice the courgettes with a mandolin or slicer . In a bowl, whisk the olive oil, lemon juice, garlic, salt and pepper. Pour the dressing over the zucchini and toss to coat. Arrange the courgettes on a serving platter and sprinkle with the goat's cheese. Garnish with fresh basil and serve.

BOILED EGGS WRAPPED IN HAM

Preparation time: 10 minutes

Cooking time: 10 minutes

Servings: 4 people

Ingredients:

4 large eggs

4 slices of ham (thinly sliced)

Salt and pepper to taste

Preparation:

Step 1: Place the eggs in a saucepan and add enough water to cover them. Bring water to a boil over high heat. Step 2: Once the water boils, reduce the heat to medium and let the eggs cook for 8 to 10 minutes for hard boiled eggs. Step 3: While the eggs cook, prepare a bowl of ice water.

Once the eggs are done, carefully transfer to the ice water using a slotted spoon. Let them sit in the ice water for a few minutes to cool and stop the cooking process. Step 4: Gently tap each egg on a hard surface to crack the shell. Peel the eggs, starting from the wide end where the air pocket is, and remove the shell. Step 5: Take a slice of ham and wrap it around each hard-boiled egg, making sure the egg is completely covered. Repeat this step for all eggs. Step 6: Season the wrapped eggs with salt and pepper to taste. If desired, you can garnish with fresh herbs such as parsley or chives. Step 7: Serve the hard-boiled eggs wrapped in ham as an appetizer or snack. They can be enjoyed hot or cold. That's all! You have your hard boiled eggs wrapped in ham ready to serve.

GRILLED PRAWNS

Preparation time: 15 minutes

Cooking time: 5-7 minutes

Servings: 4 people

Ingredients:

450g prawns, shelled and shelled

2 tablespoons of olive oil

2 cloves garlic, minced

1 tablespoon lemon juice

1 teaspoon paprika

1/2 teaspoon salt

1/4 teaspoon black pepper

Lemon wedges to serve

Preparation: Step 1: Preheat grill to medium-high heat.

Step 2: In a bowl, combine olive oil, minced garlic, lemon juice, paprika, salt and black pepper . Mix well. Step 3: Add the shrimp to the bowl and toss them in the marinade until they are evenly coated. Let them marinate for about 10 minutes. Step 4: Thread the marinated prawns onto the skewers, making sure they are spaced well apart. Step 5: Place the shrimp skewers on the preheated grill and cook for 2-3 minutes per side, or until pink and opaque. Avoid overcooking them as it can make the shrimp tough. Step 6: Once cooked, remove the prawn skewers from the grill and transfer them to a serving plate. Step 7: Garnish with fresh parsley if desired and serve the grilled shrimp hot with lemon wedges on the side. That's all! You have your delicious grilled shrimp ready to enjoy. Serve as an appetizer along with your favorite dips or salads.

AVOCADO AND SHRIMP SALAD

Preparation time: 15 minutes

Cooking time: 5 minutes

Servings: 4 people

Ingredients:

450 g of cooked prawns ,

peeled and shelled

2 ripe avocados, diced

1 cup cherry tomatoes, halved

1/2 red onion, thinly sliced

1/4 cup fresh cilantro, chopped

2 tablespoons lime juice

2 tablespoons of olive oil

Salt and pepper to taste

Optional: 1 jalapeno pepper, seeded
and chopped for added heat

Preparation:

Step 1: In a large bowl, combine the cooked shrimp, diced avocados, cherry tomatoes, red onion and cilantro . Step 2: In a separate small bowl, whisk together the lime juice, olive oil, salt, and pepper. If desired, add chopped jalapeno for a little heat. Step 3: Pour the dressing over the shrimp and avocado mixture and toss gently to evenly coat all the ingredients. Step 4: Adjust seasoning with additional salt and pepper if needed. Step 5: Let the salad sit for a few minutes to allow the flavors to meld together. Step 6: Serve the avocado and shrimp salad as a refreshing appetizer. If you wish, you can garnish it with more coriander leaves.

EGGS STUFFED WITH TUNA AND MAYONNAISE

Preparation time: 15 minutes

Cooking time: 10 minutes

Servings: 6 stuffed eggs

Ingredients:

6 hard boiled eggs

1 can tuna, drained

1/4 cup mayonnaise

1 tablespoon Dijon mustard

2 tablespoons finely chopped red onion

2 tablespoons chopped fresh parsley

Salt and pepper to taste

Optional: paprika or

fresh herbs for garnish

Preparation:

Step 1: Cut the hard-boiled eggs in half lengthwise. Carefully remove the egg yolks and place them in a bowl. Step 2: Mash the egg yolks with a fork until crumbly. Step 3: Add the drained tuna, mayonnaise, Dijon mustard, chopped red onion and chopped parsley to the bowl with the egg yolks. Mix well until all ingredients are combined. Step 4: Season the mixture with salt and pepper to taste. Adjust seasonings to your preferences. Step 5: Pour the tuna and mayonnaise mixture into the scooped out egg white halves , dividing it evenly between them. Step 6: Optional: Sprinkle the stuffed eggs with a pinch of paprika or garnish with fresh herbs such as parsley or dill. Step 7:

Place the stuffed eggs on a serving plate and refrigerate for at least 30 minutes to allow the flavors to meld together and the filling to set. Step 8: Serve the eggs stuffed with tuna and mayonnaise as an appetizer or as part of a light meal. They can be enjoyed cold. That's all! Here are your tasty Eggs Stuffed with Tuna and Mayonnaise ready to be served. Enjoy this tasty, protein-rich dish!

RAW VEGETABLE PINZIMONIO WITH CREAM CHEESE SAUCE

Preparation time: 15 minutes

Cooking time: (no cooking required)

Servings: 4 people

Ingredients:

Assorted raw vegetables such as carrots ,

celery, peppers, radishes, cherry tomatoes ,

etc., cut into sticks or pieces

For the cream cheese sauce:

1/2 cup cream cheese

1 tablespoon lemon juice

1 tablespoon extra virgin olive oil

1 clove garlic, minced

Salt and pepper to taste

Preparation:

Step 1: Prepare the raw vegetables by washing them, peeling them (if necessary) and cutting them into sticks or pieces. Step 2: In a small bowl, combine the cream cheese, lemon juice, extra virgin olive oil, minced garlic, salt and pepper. Mix well until you obtain a smooth and creamy mixture. Step 3: Arrange the prepared raw vegetables on a platter or individual serving plates. Step 4: Serve the raw vegetables with the cream cheese sauce on the side as a dip or drizzle the sauce over the vegetables. Step 5: Optional: Garnish with fresh herbs such as parsley or chives for added flavor and presentation. That's all! You have your refreshing raw vegetable dip with cream cheese sauce ready to enjoy.

AUBERGINES ROLLS WITH CHEESE AND TOMATO

Preparation time: 20 minutes

Cooking time: 20 minutes

Servings: 4-6 sandwiches

Ingredients:

1 large aubergine

Olive oil for brushing

Salt and pepper to taste

1 cup cottage cheese

1/4 grated parmesan

1/4 cup chopped fresh basil

1 cup marinara sauce (store-bought or homemade)

Preparation:

Step 1: Preheat the oven to 190°C. Step 2: Slice the eggplant lengthwise into thin slices, about 1/4 inch thick. Step 3: Brush both sides of the eggplant slices with olive oil and season with salt and pepper. Step 4: Place the eggplant slices on a baking sheet and bake in the preheated oven for about 10 to 12 minutes or until tender and pliable. Step 5: In a bowl, combine the ricotta, grated parmesan and chopped fresh basil. Mix well. Step 6: Remove the cooked eggplant slices from the oven and let them cool slightly. Step 7: Pour a dollop of the ricotta mixture onto each eggplant slice and spread it evenly. Step 8:

Roll each aubergine slice tightly and place on a baking tray, seam side down. Step 9: Pour the marinara sauce over the eggplant wraps, covering them evenly. Step 10: Optional: Sprinkle some grated Parmesan cheese over the rolls. Step 11: Bake the eggplant rolls in the preheated oven for about 10 minutes, or until heated through and the cheese is melted and bubbly. Step 12: Serve the eggplant rolls with cheese and tomato as an appetizer. They can be enjoyed hot.

SMOKED SALMON WITH CUCUMBER AND CREAM OF CHEESE

Preparation time: 10 minutes

Cooking time: no cooking

Servings: 4 people

Ingredients:

8 slices of smoked salmon

1 cucumber, thinly sliced

Cheese cream

Fresh dill or chives for garnish (optional)

Lemon wedges to serve

Preparation:

Step 1: Arrange the smoked salmon slices on a serving platter or individual plates. Step 2: Place a slice of cucumber on each slice of smoked salmon. Step 3: Spread a dollop of cream cheese over the cucumber slices. Step 4: Optional: Garnish with fresh dill or chives for added flavor and presentation. Step 5: Serve the smoked salmon with cucumber and cream cheese as an appetizer or light snack, accompanied by lemon wedges to squeeze over the salmon.

MOZZARELLA BALLS WITH TOMATO AND BASIL

Preparation time: 15 minutes

Cooking time: (no cooking required)

Servings: 4 people

Ingredients:

200 g of buffalo mozzarella

2 ripe tomatoes

Fresh basil leaves

salt

Pepper

Extra virgin olive oil

Preparation:

Start by cutting the mozzarella into equal-sized cubes. Also cut the cherry tomatoes into cubes the same size as the mozzarella pieces. Take a fresh basil leaf and place it on top of a piece of mozzarella. Wrap the basil around the cheese, creating a sphere. Repeat the process for all the mozzarella. Now take a spherical piece of mozzarella and wrap it with a piece of tomato. Use your fingers to lightly press the edges to seal the ball. Repeat the process for all the mozzarella balls. Arrange the mozzarella with the tomato on a serving plate. Season with salt, pepper and a drizzle of extra virgin olive oil. Decorate with a few fresh basil leaves. Serve the mozzarella with tomatoes and basil immediately and enjoy them while they are fresh.

BEEF CARPACCIO WITH ARUGULA AND PARMESAN

Preparation time: approximately 15 minutes.

Cooking Times: No time since

the dish should be served raw.

Doses for 4 people:

Ingredients:

300 g of beef fillet.

240 g of arugula.

200 g of grated parmesan.

Juice of 2 lemons.

Extra virgin olive oil.

Salt and freshly ground black pepper.

Preparation:

Lightly freeze the beef tenderloin to make cutting easier. Then slice it thinly with a sharp knife. Arrange the beef slices on a serving plate. Season with lemon juice, olive oil, salt and black pepper. Distribute the arugula evenly over the meat. Sprinkle the grated Parmesan generously over the carpaccio. Serve immediately and enjoy it as a fresh and light appetizer.

GRILLED CHICKEN SALAD WITH MAYONNAISE

Preparation time: 20-30 minutes.

Cooking times: 10-15 minutes

Doses for 4 people:

Ingredients:

500 g of chicken breast.

800 g of mixed salad.

2 ripe tomatoes.

2 cucumbers.

2 carrots.

2 red peppers.

16 tablespoons of mayonnaise.

Juice of 2 lemons.

Olive oil to taste Salt and pepper to taste.

Preparation:

Grill the chicken breast until cooked through and golden brown. Let it cool, then cut it into cubes. Dice the tomatoes, cucumbers, carrots and peppers. In a large bowl, add the lettuce mix, tomatoes, cucumbers, carrots, peppers and grilled chicken. Season with mayonnaise, lemon juice, olive oil, salt and pepper. Mix well to combine all the ingredients. Serve grilled chicken salad with mayonnaise as a main course or as a side dish. You can add some toasted croutons to go with it if you like.

SMOKED SALMON CANAPES WITH CREAM CHEESE

Preparation time: 10-15 minutes.

Cooking times: none

Doses for 4 people:

Ingredients:

8 slices of bread.

200 g of smoked salmon.

150g cream cheese.

Juice of 1 lemon.

Fresh chives to taste

Salt and freshly ground

black pepper to taste

Preparation:

In a bowl, mix the cream cheese with the lemon juice, chopped chives, salt and pepper. Mix until you obtain a smooth and well-blended cream. Lightly toast the bread slices. Spread a generous amount of cream cheese on each slice of toast. Cut the smoked salmon into strips or smaller pieces and place it on the cream cheese. Garnish with fresh chives and black pepper. Serve the smoked salmon canapé with cream cheese as an appetizer.

RAW HAM WITH MELON

Preparation time: 10 minutes.

Cooking times: none.

Ingredients:

Doses for 4 people:

8 slices of raw ham.

1 ripe melon.

Fresh mint leaves to taste

Freshly ground black

pepper (optional).

Preparation:

Cut the melon in half and remove the seeds. Remove the peel and cut the pulp into slices or wedges. Wrap each slice of melon with a slice of raw ham. Arrange the slices of raw ham with the melon on a serving plate. Garnish with a few fresh mint leaves. If you like, you can add a pinch of freshly ground black pepper to flavor everything. Serve the raw ham with melon as an appetizer or summer snack.

GRILLED CHICKEN SKEWERS WITH PEPPERS

Preparation time: approximately 20-30 minutes.

Cooking times: approximately 10-15 minutes.

Doses for 4 people:

Ingredients:

4 chicken breasts.

2 peppers (preferably

of different colors) .

Extra virgin olive oil.

Juice of 1 lemon.

Salt and pepper to taste.

Preparation:

Preheat grill to medium-high heat. Thread the chicken and pepper cubes alternately onto the skewers. Season the skewers with olive oil, lemon juice, salt and pepper. Place the skewers on the grill and cook for about 10-15 minutes, turning occasionally, until the chicken is cooked through and the peppers are soft and lightly browned. Remove the skewers from the grill and let them rest for a few minutes before serving. Serve the grilled chicken skewers with peppers as a second course accompanied by side dishes of your choice.

LIVER PATÉ WITH CELERY CROUTTONS

Preparation time: 20-30 minutes.

Cooking times: 10-15 minutes.

Doses for 4 people:

Ingredients:

250 g of chicken or veal liver.

1 medium onion, chopped.

2 cloves garlic, minced.

50 g of butter.

2 tablespoons of olive oil.

50 ml of dry white wine.

Salt and pepper.

Celery, cut into sticks, for crostini.

Preparation:

In a skillet, melt the butter with the olive oil over medium-high heat. Add the chopped onion and garlic and cook until soft and golden. Add the chicken or calf liver to the pan and cook for about 5 to 7 minutes, until cooked through but still soft . Deglaze with dry white wine and let the alcohol evaporate. Transfer everything into the bowl of a blender or immersion blender and blend until you obtain a smooth and homogeneous mixture. Season with salt and pepper according to your taste. Prepare celery croutons by cutting the celery into sticks and spreading the liver pâté on top. Serve the liver pâté with celery croutons as an appetizer or snack.

OLIVES STUFFED WITH CHEESE

Preparation time: approximately 15 minutes.

Cooking times: none

Doses for 4 people:

Ingredients:

pitted green olives .

100 g of cheese (of your choice).

Freshly ground black pepper (optional).

Preparation:

Drain and rinse the olives well to remove the preservation liquid. Take a small amount of cheese and gently stuff each olive. Continue filling all the olives with cheese. If you like, you can sprinkle the stuffed olives with freshly ground black pepper to add flavour. Serve the cheese-stuffed olives as an appetizer.

CANNED MACKEREL WITH AVOCADO AND LIME

Preparation time: approximately 10 minutes.

Cooking times: none.

Doses for 4 people:

Ingredients:

2 cans of canned mackerel.

2 ripe avocados.

Juice of 2 limes.

Salt and freshly ground black pepper.

Preparation:

Drain the oil or preserving liquid from the canned mackerel. In a bowl, crumble the mackerel with a fork. Add the avocado slices and lime juice to the bowl with the crumbled mackerel. Gently mix the ingredients until well combined. Season with salt and pepper to your taste. Serve canned mackerel with avocado and lime as a salad or spread on slices of toast as bruschetta.

STUFFED COURGETTES WITH MINCED MEAT

Preparation time: 20 minutes.

Cooking times: 30-40 minutes.

Doses for 4 people:

Ingredients:

4 medium sized courgettes.

300 g of minced meat.

1 onion.

2 cloves of garlic.

1 red pepper , 1 carrot.

200 g of peeled tomatoes.

Grated Parmesan cheese.

Salt and pepper to taste. Olive oil.

Preparation:

Preheat the oven to 180°C. Cut the courgettes in half lengthwise and delicately remove the central pulp. In a pan, heat a drizzle of oil and add the chopped onion and garlic. Fry until golden brown. Add the ground beef to the pan and cook until well browned. Add the pepper and carrot cut into cubes and continue cooking for a few minutes. Add the peeled tomatoes cut into pieces, salt and pepper. Mix well and cook for 10-15 minutes. Fill the empty courgettes with the prepared meat filling. Arrange the stuffed courgettes on a baking tray lightly greased with olive oil. Sprinkle the grated cheese over the zucchini. Bake in the preheated oven for about 20 to 25 minutes, or until the courgettes are tender and the cheese is golden and melted. Serve the stuffed courgettes with minced meat.

BROCCOLI AND CHEESE FLAN

Preparation time: 20 minutes

Cooking times: 40 minutes

ingredients:

Doses for 4 people:

500 g of fresh broccoli

200 g of grated cheese

4 eggs

200 ml of milk

Nutmeg to taste (optional)

Preparation:

Preheat the oven to 180°C. Clean the broccoli and cut them into florets. Cook them in salted water for about 5 minutes, until they are tender.

Drain them and let them cool slightly. In a bowl, beat the eggs and add the milk. Add the grated cheese and mix well. Season with salt, pepper, and nutmeg (if desired). Add the broccoli to the egg and cheese mixture and stir gently to evenly distribute the ingredients. Pour the mixture into a buttered pan. Bake in the preheated oven for about 40 minutes or until the top is golden brown and the flan is cooked through. Remove from the oven and let rest a few minutes before serving. You can accompany the broccoli and cheese flan with a fresh green salad or crusty bread.

ROASTED PEPPER ROLLS WITH RICOTTA

Preparation time: 15 minutes

Cooking times: 25 minutes

ingredients:

Doses for 4 people:

3 peppers of different colors

200 g of ricotta

50 g of grated parmesan

1 clove garlic, minced

2 tablespoons fresh parsley, chopped

Salt and pepper to taste ., Olive oil to taste

Preparation:

Preheat the oven to 200°C. Cut the peppers in half, remove the seeds and internal white filaments.

Place them on a parchment-lined baking sheet, skin side up. Bake the peppers in the preheated oven for about 15 minutes, until the skin is lightly charred. Remove the peppers from the oven and let them cool slightly. Gently peel the skin off the roasted peppers. It will be easier to remove them now that they are warm. In a bowl mix the ricotta, grated cheese, garlic and parsley. Season with salt and pepper according to your taste. Take a roasted pepper and spread some ricotta filling on it. Roll the pepper around the filling. Repeat the process with the other peppers. Arrange the pepper rolls on a lightly oiled baking tray. Bake in the preheated oven for about 10 minutes, until the rolls are hot and lightly browned. Serve the pepper rolls.

OCTOPUS SALAD WITH CELERY AND LEMON

Preparation time: 20 minutes

Cooking times: 40 minutes

ingredients:

Doses for 4 people:

1 fresh octopus (about 1 kg)

2 stalks celery, thinly sliced

Juice of 1 lemon

3 tablespoons of extra virgin olive oil

Salt and pepper to taste.

Chopped fresh parsley (for garnish)

Preparation:

Clean the octopus by removing the head and internal organs. Rinse it well under cold water.

In a large saucepan, bring plenty of lightly salted water to the boil. Dip the octopus into the boiling water for 5 seconds, then take it out. Repeat this 2-3 more times to help tighten the skin of the octopus. Reduce the heat and place the octopus in the pot. Simmer for about 40 minutes or until tender. You can test the doneness by inserting the tip of a knife into the thickest part of the octopus: if it enters easily, it is cooked. Drain the octopus and let it cool completely. Cut the cooled octopus into pieces of the desired size. In a bowl, mix lemon juice, olive oil, salt and pepper to make a vinaigrette. Add the cut octopus and sliced celery to the bowl with the vinaigrette. Stir gently to evenly distribute the vinaigrette. Leave the octopus salad in the refrigerator for at least 30 minutes to flavor. Before serving, garnish with chopped fresh parsley.

ASPARAGUS WRAPPED IN HAM

Preparation time: 10 minutes

Cooking times: 15 minutes

Doses for 4 people:

ingredients:

16 fresh asparagus

8 slices of raw ham

Olive oil

Salt and pepper

Preparation:

Preheat the oven to 200°C. Take the fresh asparagus and wrap it with half a slice of raw ham. Repeat the operation with the other asparagus. Arrange the ham-wrapped asparagus on a lightly oiled baking tray. Drizzle the asparagus with a drizzle of olive oil and season with salt and pepper. Bake in the preheated oven for about 15 minutes or until the ham is crispy and the asparagus is tender. Remove from the oven and serve the asparagus wrapped in ham as an appetizer warm or at room temperature.

SALMON MOUSSE WITH DRIED TOMATOES

Preparation time: 20 minutes

Cooking times:

None (cold mousse)

Doses for 4 people:

ingredients:

200 g of smoked salmon

150 g of spreadable cheese

4 dried tomatoes

Juice of half a lemon

Salt and pepper to taste.

Preparation:

Cut the smoked salmon into small pieces and place in a mixer or blender. Add the spreadable cheese, the dried tomatoes soaked in hot water for a few minutes and the lemon juice. Blend everything until you obtain a creamy and homogeneous consistency. Taste and adjust salt and pepper to your taste. Transfer the salmon mousse to small bowls or glasses for presentation. Cover and place in the fridge for at least an hour to firm up the mousse. Before serving you can garnish the mousse with fresh parsley leaves or grated lemon zest. Serve the salmon mousse with dried tomatoes as an appetizer on crostini or with crackers.

GRILLED SHRIMP AND COURGETTE SKEWERS

Preparation time: 20 minutes

Cooking times: 10 minutes

Doses for 4 people:

ingredients:

16 fresh prawns, peeled and cleaned

2 medium courgettes

Juice of 1 lemon

Olive oil to taste

Salt and pepper to taste.

Preparation:

Preheat your grill or barbecue. Cut the courgettes into thin slices lengthwise. In a bowl, season the prawns with lemon juice, a drizzle of olive oil, salt and pepper. Thread the prawn and courgette slices alternately onto the skewers. Brush the skewers with a drizzle of olive oil to prevent them from sticking to the grill. Cook the skewers on the grill or barbecue for about 5 minutes per side, until the prawns are cooked through and the courgettes have nice streaks from the grill. Remove the skewers from the grill and serve them hot as an appetizer or as a main course accompanied by a fresh green salad.

BOILED EGGS STUFFED WITH GUACAMOLE

Preparation time: 15 minutes

Cooking times: 10 minutes

Doses for 4 people:

ingredients:

8 eggs

2 ripe avocados

Juice of 1 lime

1 small, ripe tomato, finely chopped

1 clove garlic, finely chopped

1 tablespoon red onion, finely chopped

Salt and pepper to taste.

Preparation:

Place the eggs in a saucepan with cold water and bring to the boil. Cook for about 10 minutes. Drain them and cool them under cold running water. Peel the eggs and cut them in half lengthwise. In a bowl, mash the avocados with a fork until you get a creamy consistency. Add the lime juice and mix well. Add the chopped tomato, garlic and red onion to the bowl with the avocado. Mix gently. Season with salt and pepper to your taste. Fill the hard-boiled egg halves with the prepared guacamole. You can garnish the guacamole-filled eggs with chopped fresh parsley or a sprinkle of sweet paprika for extra presentation. Serve hard-boiled eggs filled with guacamole as an appetizer or as finger food on special occasions.

AUBERGINES ROLLATINI WITH CHEESE AND COOKED HAM

Preparation time: 30 minutes

Cooking times: 20-25 minutes

Doses for 4 people:

ingredients:

2 medium aubergines, 200 g of sliced cheese

8 slices of raw ham

Tomato puree

Olive oil, salt and pepper

Grated Parmesan cheese

Preparation:

Preheat the oven to 180°C. Cut the aubergines into thin slices lengthwise. You can use a mandolin to get even slices.

Place the aubergine slices in a bowl and season them with a little salt. Let them rest for about 10 minutes to release excess water. Then, rinse them under cold water and pat dry with a clean towel. Distribute a slice of cheese and a slice of ham on each slice of aubergine. Gently roll up the aubergine slices with the cheese and ham inside. Repeat the process with all the aubergine slices. Take a baking tray and spread a little tomato puree on the bottom. Arrange the aubergine rolls in the pan, with the rolled side facing down. Season the rollatini with a drizzle of oil, salt and pepper. Sprinkle some grated cheese on top. Bake in the preheated oven for about 20-25 minutes, until the rollatini are golden and the cheese melted . Remove from the oven and let rest a few minutes before serving.

COOKED HAM WITH SLICES OF CHEESE

Preparation time: 5 minutes

Cooking times:

None (cold dish)

Doses for 4 people:

ingredients:

8 slices of cooked ham

8 slices of cheese

Preparation:

Take a slice of cooked ham and place a slice of cheese in the center. Roll the slice of ham around the slice of cheese, creating a roll. Repeat the process with the other slices of cooked ham and cheese. You can serve cooked hams with slices of cheese as a cold appetizer or as part of a charcuterie board.

SWORDFISH CARPACCIO WITH CITRUS FRUITS

Preparation time: 15 minutes

Cooking times: None (raw dish)

Doses for 4 people:

ingredients:

400 g of fresh swordfish fillet

Juice of 2 lemons

Juice of 1 orange

Grated zest of 1 lemon

Grated zest of 1 orange

Extra virgin olive oil

Salt and pepper

Rocket or mixed salad

Preparation:

Cut the swordfish fillet into thin slices and arrange them on a serving plate. In a bowl, mix together the lemon juice, orange juice and grated lemon and orange zest. Pour the citrus dressing over the swordfish slices, taking care to cover all the slices well. Leave to marinate for about 10 minutes. Add a drizzle of extra virgin olive oil to the swordfish carpaccio and season with salt and pepper. Garnish with arugula or fresh mixed salad. Serve the swordfish carpaccio with citrus fruits as an appetizer or as a light dish.

CHICKEN ROLLS WITH HAM AND CHEESE

Preparation time: 20 minutes

Cooking times: 25-30 minutes

Doses for 4 people:

ingredients:

4 chicken breasts

8 slices of raw ham

8 slices of cheese

Olive oil

Salt and pepper

Preparation:

Preheat the oven to 180°C. Take a chicken breast and cut it in half lengthwise. Lightly flatten each half with a meat mallet. Arrange a slice of ham and a slice of cheese on the flattened chicken breast. Wrap the chicken breast around the ham and cheese and secure with a toothpick. Repeat the process with the other chicken breasts. Heat a non-stick pan with a drizzle of oil and brown the chicken rolls on all sides until golden. Transfer the chicken rolls to a baking sheet and bake in the preheated oven for about 15-20 minutes, or until the chicken is cooked through. Remove from the oven and let rest a few minutes before serving.

MIXED VEGETABLE OMELETTE

Preparation time: 15 minutes

Cooking times: 15-20 minutes

Doses for 4 people:

ingredients:

6 eggs

1 medium courgette, diced

1 red pepper, diced

1 medium onion, diced

100 g button mushrooms, sliced

Grated parmesan to taste

Olive oil to taste

Salt and pepper to taste.

Preparation:

In a non-stick pan, heat a drizzle of oil and add the onion. Cook until soft and translucent. Add the zucchini, bell pepper and mushrooms to the pan. Cook vegetables until tender. In a bowl, beat the eggs and add the cooked vegetables. Mix well. Season with salt, pepper and grated cheese to taste. Heat some olive oil in a larger pan and pour the egg and vegetable mixture into the pan. E. Cook the omelette over medium-low heat for about 10 to 15 minutes or until the bottom is golden brown and the top is done. Flip the omelette onto a flat plate and then return it to the pan to cook the other side for a few minutes. Remove from the pan and leave to cool for a few minutes before cutting into wedges. Garnish with chopped fresh parsley and serve the mixed vegetable omelette as a second course or side dish.

BRUSCHETTE WITH TOMATO AND BASIL

Preparation time: 10 minutes

Cooking times: 5-7 minutes

Doses for 4 people:

ingredients:

4 slices of rustic bread

(Tuscan bread or ciabatta)

2 ripe tomatoes, diced

Fresh basil leaves, to taste

1 clove of garlic, cut in half

Extra virgin olive oil to taste

Salt and pepper to taste.

Preparation:

Preheat the oven to 180°C. Place the bread slices on a baking tray and toast them in the preheated oven for about 5-7 minutes or until crispy. Rub the surface of the bread slices with the halved garlic to impart a light flavor. In a bowl, mix the diced tomatoes with the fresh basil. Season with salt, pepper and a drizzle of extra virgin olive oil. Spread the tomato and basil mixture over the toasted bread slices. You can add more fresh basil leaves as a garnish. Serve the bruschetta with tomato and basil as an appetizer or as a tasty snack.

TUNA SALAD WITH BOILED EGGS AND OLIVES

Preparation time: 15 minutes

Cooking times: 10 minutes

Doses for 4 people:

ingredients:

2 cans of tuna

canned (drained)

4 eggs

pitted black olives

1 cucumber, diced

1 red pepper, diced

1 tomato, diced

Juice of 1 lemon

Extra virgin olive oil to taste

Salt and pepper to taste.

Preparation:

In a saucepan, bring lightly salted water to the boil. Add the eggs and cook them for about 10 minutes to obtain hard-boiled eggs. Drain them and let them cool before peeling them and cutting them in half. In a bowl, mix the drained tuna, olives, cucumber, pepper and diced tomato. Add the lemon juice, a drizzle of extra virgin olive oil, salt and pepper. Mix well to combine all the ingredients. Add the halved hard-boiled eggs to the bowl with the other ingredients or place them on top of the salad. Serve the tuna salad with hard-boiled eggs and olives as a second course or as an appetizer.

CHEESE AND SPECK POUCHES

Preparation time: 15 minutes

Cooking times: 15-20 minutes

Doses for 4 people:

ingredients:

1 roll of pasta

rectangular sheet

100 g of sliced cheese

100 g of sliced speck

1 egg

Sesame seeds or

poppy (optional)

Preparation:

Preheat the oven to 180°C. Unroll the puff pastry and cut it into strips about 2-3 cm wide. Take a strip of puff pastry and wrap a slice of cheese and a slice of speck inside. Continue the process until the ingredients are used up. Place the puff pastries on a baking tray lined with baking paper. Brush the sheets with the beaten egg to give them an even browning. If desired, you can sprinkle sesame or poppy seeds on the puff pastry. Bake in the preheated oven for about 15-20 minutes, or until the sheets are golden and crispy . Remove from the oven and let cool slightly before serving the cheese and speck puff pastries as an appetizer or starter.

MEATBALLS WITH CHEESE SAUCE

Preparation time: 20 minutes

Cooking times: 25-30 minutes

Doses for 4 people:

ingredients:

500 g of minced meat

1 egg

1/2 cup breadcrumbs

1/4 grated parmesan

1 clove of garlic

1 tablespoon fresh parsley

Salt and pepper, olive oil

1 cup cheese sauce

Preparation:

In a bowl, mix the minced meat with the egg, breadcrumbs, grated cheese, chopped garlic, parsley, salt and pepper. Work the ingredients until you obtain a homogeneous mixture. Take a portion of the meat mixture and shape it into evenly sized meatballs. Heat a drizzle of olive oil in a pan and cook the meatballs over medium-high heat until browned on all sides and cooked through. It will take about 10-15 minutes. Meanwhile, heat the cheese sauce in a saucepan over medium-low heat. Transfer the cooked meatballs to the pot with the cheese sauce and toss gently to coat completely. Continue cooking for a few minutes to allow the meatballs to absorb the cheese sauce. Serve the meatballs with cheese sauce as a second course, accompanied by side dishes of your choice.

SALMON CANAPES WITH CUCUMBER AND AVOCADO

Preparation time: 15 minutes

Cooking times: None (cold dish)

Doses for 4 people:

ingredients:

4 slices of bread (wholemeal bread or baguette)

200 g smoked salmon, cut into slices

1 cucumber, thinly sliced

1 ripe avocado, sliced

Lemon juice

Salt and pepper to taste.

Chives or fresh dill (for garnish)

Preparation:

Lightly toast the bread slices. Arrange the toasted bread slices on a plate. Place a slice of smoked salmon, a few slices of cucumber and a few slices of avocado on each slice of bread . Squeeze some lemon juice over the salmon, cucumber and avocado to prevent oxidation of the avocado and add salt and pepper to taste. Garnish the canapés with chives or fresh dill. Serve the salmon canapés with cucumber and avocado as an appetizer or as a tasty snack.

MOZZARELLA IN CARROZZA WITHOUT BREAD

Preparation time: 15 minutes

Cooking times: 10-15 minutes

Doses for 4 people:

ingredients:

2 fresh buffalo mozzarella

Flour

2 eggs

Bread crumbs

Peanut oil

Salt and pepper

Tomato sauce

or marinara sauce

Preparation:

Cut the mozzarella into slices about 1 cm thick. Prepare three bowls: one with the flour, one with the beaten eggs and one with the breadcrumbs. Dip the mozzarella slices in the flour, then in the beaten egg, and finally in the breadcrumbs, making the breadcrumbs adhere well on both sides. Heat plenty of peanut oil in a non-stick pan. Fry the breaded mozzarella in hot oil until golden brown on both sides, about 2-3 minutes per side. Drain them on absorbent paper to remove excess oil. Season freshly fried with salt and pepper and serve hot with tomato sauce or marinara sauce for dipping.

EGGS STUFFED WITH SALMON AND SPREADABLE CHEESE

Preparation time: 20 minutes

Cooking times: 10 minutes

Doses for 4 people:

ingredients:

8 eggs

100 g of smoked salmon ,

cut into small pieces

4 tablespoons cream cheese

(e.g. Philadelphia)

Lemon juice

Salt and pepper to taste.

Chives or parsley

fresh, chopped (for garnish)

Preparation:

Bring a pot of water to a boil. Add the eggs and cook them for about 10 minutes to obtain hard-boiled eggs. Drain them and let them cool before peeling them. Cut the eggs in half lengthwise and gently remove the yolks. Place the egg yolks in a bowl. Mash the egg yolks with a fork and add the smoked salmon cut into pieces, the cream cheese and a little lemon juice. Mix well until you obtain a creamy consistency. Season with salt and pepper. Fill the egg halves with the yolk and salmon mixture. E. Garnish with chives or chopped fresh parsley. Serve stuffed eggs with salmon and cream cheese as an appetizer or as finger food on special occasions.

HAM AND ASPARAGUS ROLLS

Preparation time: 15 minutes

Cooking times: 10-15 minutes

Doses for 4 people:

ingredients:

16 fresh asparagus

8 slices of raw ham

Olive oil

Salt and pepper

Preparation:

Preheat the oven to 200°C. Cut the woody part of the asparagus and rinse them. Bring a pan of lightly salted water to the boil.

Add the asparagus and cook for about 3-4 minutes, until tender but still crunchy . Drain them and pass them under cold water to stop the cooking. Take a slice of raw ham and wrap two asparagus in it, so that the ham completely envelops the asparagus. Repeat the process with the remaining slices of ham and asparagus. Arrange the ham and asparagus rolls on a baking tray lined with baking paper. Brush the rolls lightly with olive oil, salt and pepper to taste. Bake in the preheated oven for about 10-15 minutes, until the ham is crispy. Remove from the oven and let rest for a few minutes before serving the ham and asparagus rolls as an appetizer or side dish.

AVOCADO AND CHICKEN SALAD WITH YOGURT SAUCE

Preparation time: 20 minutes

Cooking times: 15-20 minutes

Doses for 4 people:

ingredients:

2 chicken breasts, grilled and cut into strips

2 ripe avocados, cut into slices

2 cups mixed lettuce, washed and chopped

1 cucumber, thinly sliced

1/2 red onion, thinly sliced

Juice of 1 lemon

1/2 cup Greek yogurt

1 clove garlic, finely chopped

Chopped fresh chives or parsley (for garnish)

Salt and pepper to taste.

Preparation:

Grill the chicken breasts until cooked through. Let them cool slightly, then cut them into strips. In a bowl, combine grilled chicken, sliced avocado, lettuce, cucumber, and sliced red onion. In another bowl, prepare the sauce by mixing the Greek yogurt, lemon juice, chopped garlic, salt and pepper. Mix well to obtain a creamy sauce. Pour the yogurt sauce over the chicken and vegetable mixture and toss gently to coat evenly. Garnish with chives or chopped fresh parsley. Serve Avocado Chicken Salad with Yogurt Dressing as a main course or as a light salad.

ARTICHOKE AND CHEESE FLAN

Preparation time: 20 minutes

Cooking times: 30-35 minutes

Doses for 4 people:

ingredients:

4 fresh artichokes

200 g of grated cheese

(for example, pecorino or parmesan)

4 eggs

200 ml of fresh cream

Salt and pepper to taste.

Butter to grease the pan

Preparation:

Prepare the artichokes: remove the tough outer leaves, cut off the top of the artichokes and cut off the base. Remove leaf tips if necessary. Cut the artichokes in half and remove the internal hay. Boil the artichokes in boiling salted water for about 10-15 minutes or until tender. Drain them and let them cool slightly. Preheat the oven to 180°C. Butter a baking tray. In a bowl, beat the eggs and add the fresh cream. Add the grated cheese and mix well. Season with salt and pepper to taste. Place the artichokes in the buttered pan and pour the egg and cheese mixture over them. Bake in the preheated oven for about 20-25 minutes, or until the top is golden brown and the pie is firm. Remove from the oven and leave to cool before serving the artichoke and cheese flan as a second course or side dish.

PAN-FED PRAWNS WITH GARLIC AND PARSLEY

Preparation time: 10 minutes

Cooking times: 5-7 minutes

Doses for 4 people:

ingredients:

500g fresh prawns, peeled

and deprived of the intestines

4 tablespoons of olive oil

4 cloves garlic, finely chopped

Fresh parsley,

chopped to taste

Salt and pepper to taste.

Preparation:

Rinse the prawns under cold running water and dry them with absorbent paper. In a nonstick skillet, heat the olive oil over medium-high heat. Add the chopped garlic cloves and cook for a few minutes, until lightly browned and fragrant. Add the prawns to the pan and cook for about 3-4 minutes on each side, until pink and cooked through. Season with salt and pepper to taste during cooking. Remove the pan from the heat and sprinkle the prawns with chopped fresh parsley. Serve the scampi in a pan with garlic and parsley as an appetizer or as a second course, perhaps accompanied by some croutons.

RECIPES
FIRST DISHES

CABBAGE AND SAUSAGE SOUP

Preparation time: 20 minutes

Cooking time: 30 minutes

Doses for: 4 people

Ingredients:

200 g onion, chopped

2 cloves garlic, minced

2 tablespoons olive oil

500 g savoy cabbage, chopped

1 liter vegetable broth

400 g peeled tomatoes, undrained

1 teaspoon dried oregano

1/2 teaspoon black pepper

400 g sweet Italian sausage, crumbled

Salt to taste

Preparation:

Saute the onion and garlic in olive oil until soft. Add the savoy cabbage and cook for 5 minutes. Pour in the vegetable broth, peeled tomatoes, oregano and black pepper. Bring to the boil and simmer for 20 minutes. Add the crumbled sausage and cook for another 5 minutes. Taste and adjust seasonings to taste. Serve hot with crusty bread.

ZUCCHINI TAGLIATELLE WITH TOMATO SAUCE AND MEATBALLS

Preparation time: 20 minutes

Cooking times: 30 minutes

Ingredients:

Serves 4 people

4 courgettes

500 g of minced meat

1 onion, chopped

2 cloves garlic, minced

400 g of tomato puree

1 tablespoon olive oil

1 teaspoon dried oregano

Salt and pepper to taste.

Preparation:

Cut the courgettes into julienne strips to obtain courgette "tagliatelle". In a pan, heat the olive oil and add the onion and garlic. Fry until golden. Add the ground beef to the pan and cook until well browned. Add the tomato puree, oregano, salt and pepper. Mix well and cook over medium-low heat for about 15-20 minutes. Meanwhile, in a separate pan, cook the courgette tagliatelle for 2-3 minutes until tender. Serve the courgette tagliatelle with the tomato sauce and meatballs on top. Enjoy your meal!

AUBERGINES LASAGNE WITHOUT PASTA

Preparation time: 30 minutes

Cooking times: 40 minutes

Ingredients:

Serves 4 people

2 large aubergines

400 g of minced meat

1 onion, chopped, 2 cloves garlic, chopped

400 g of tomato puree

250g mozzarella, sliced

50 g of grated cheese

1 tablespoon olive oil

Salt and pepper to taste.

Preparation:

Cut the aubergines into thin slices and grill them until soft. In a pan, heat the olive oil and add the onion and garlic. Fry until golden. Add the ground beef to the pan and cook until well browned. Add the tomato puree, salt and pepper. Mix well and cook over medium-low heat for about 15 minutes. In a pan, start creating the layers by alternating the aubergine slices, the ragù and the mozzarella. Continue alternating layers until you run out of ingredients, making sure to finish with a layer of mozzarella on top. Sprinkle the grated cheese over the lasagna. Bake in a preheated oven at 180°C for approximately 25-30 minutes or until the cheese is golden and melted. Let it rest for a few minutes before serving. Enjoy your meal!

ZUCCHINI SPAGHETTI WITH AVOCADO PESTO

Preparation time: 15 minutes

Cooking times: none

The ingredients:

Serves 4 people

4 courgettes, 1 ripe avocado

1 bunch of fresh basil

1 clove of garlic

Juice of 1 lemon

30 g of almonds or pine nuts

3 tablespoons of olive oil

Salt and pepper to taste.

Preparation:

Cut the courgettes into julienne strips or use a spiral to create courgette spaghetti. In a food processor or blender, combine the avocado, basil, garlic clove, lemon juice, almonds or pine nuts, olive oil, salt and pepper. Blend until you obtain a creamy consistency. Toss the avocado pesto with the zucchini noodles until well seasoned. Serve the courgette spaghetti with the avocado pesto. Enjoy your meal!

TOMATO SOUP WITH CHICKEN AND VEGETABLES

Preparation time: 20 minutes

Cooking times: 30 minutes

Ingredients:

Serves 4 people

2 chicken breasts, cut into cubes

1 onion, chopped

2 carrots, cut into rounds

2 stalks celery, cut into slices

3 cloves garlic, minced

800 g peeled tomatoes, chopped

1 liter of chicken broth

1 teaspoon dried oregano

1 teaspoon dried basil

Salt and pepper to taste.

Olive oil for cooking

Preparation:

In a large pot, heat a drizzle of olive oil and add the onion, carrots, celery and garlic. Fry until golden. Add the diced chicken to the pot and cook until golden brown. Add chopped canned tomatoes, chicken broth, oregano, basil, salt and pepper. Mix well and bring to the boil. Reduce the heat and cook over medium-low heat for about 20 to 25 minutes, or until the chicken is cooked through and the vegetables are tender. Taste and adjust salt and pepper, if necessary. Serve the tomato soup with chicken and vegetables hot . Enjoy your meal!

CUCUMBER NOODLES WITH TUNA AND AVOCADO SAUCE

Preparation time: 15 minutes

Cooking times: none

Ingredients:

Serves 4 people

2 cucumbers

2 cans of drained tuna

1 ripe avocado

Juice of 1 lemon

1 tablespoon olive oil

1 red onion, thinly sliced

Chopped fresh parsley to taste

Salt and pepper to taste.

Preparation:

Using a vegetable peeler, create cucumber "noodles." Set them aside. In a bowl, mash the avocado until you get a creamy consistency. Add the lemon juice, olive oil, salt and pepper. Mix well to obtain the avocado sauce. In another bowl, combine the drained tuna, red onion and chopped parsley. Stir gently to season the tuna. Add the cucumber "noodles" to the avocado sauce and stir to evenly distribute the sauce. Arrange the cucumber tagliatelle on a serving platter and garnish with the seasoned tuna on top. Serve the cucumber noodles with tuna and avocado sauce. Enjoy your meal!

PRAWNS SALAD WITH AVOCADO AND LIME

Preparation time: 20 minutes

Cooking times: 5 minutes

Ingredients:

Serves 4 people

500 g of peeled prawns

2 ripe avocados, diced, Juice of 2 limes

1 cucumber, cut into thin slices

1 red pepper, diced

1 red onion, thinly sliced

Chopped fresh parsley to taste

Olive oil for cooking prawns

Salt and pepper to taste.

Preparation:

In a pan, heat a drizzle of olive oil and cook the peeled prawns until pink and cooked through, about 3-5 minutes. In a large bowl, combine the diced avocados, lime juice, thinly sliced cucumber, diced red bell pepper and red onion. Stir gently to season the ingredients. Add the cooked shrimp to the salad and toss lightly. Season with salt and pepper according to your taste. Sprinkle the salad with chopped fresh parsley. Serve the shrimp salad with avocado and lime. Enjoy your meal!

CAULIFLOWER RICE WITH PAN-SAUTERED VEGETABLES

Preparation time: 15 minutes

Cooking times: 15 minutes

Ingredients:

Serves 4 people

1 large cauliflower

1 courgette, cut into cubes

1 red pepper, diced

1 carrot, diced, 1 onion, chopped

2 cloves garlic, minced

2 tablespoons of olive oil

Salt and pepper to taste.

Chopped fresh parsley to taste

Preparation:

Cut the cauliflower into small pieces and put it in a mixer or blender. Blend until you get a rice-like consistency. In a large skillet, heat the olive oil and add the onion and garlic. Fry until golden. Add the vegetables (courgette, pepper and carrot) to the pan and sauté for 5-7 minutes, until tender but still crunchy . Add the grated cauliflower to the pan and mix well with the sautéed vegetables. Continue cooking for another 5 minutes. Taste and adjust salt and pepper to your taste. Serve the cauliflower rice with sautéed vegetables, garnished with chopped fresh parsley. Enjoy your meal!

ZUCCHINI SPAGHETTI WITH MEAT SAUCE

Preparation time: 20 minutes

Cooking times: 30 minutes

Ingredients:

Serves 4 people

4 courgettes

500 g of minced meat

1 onion, chopped

2 cloves garlic, minced

400 g of tomato puree

1 tablespoon olive oil

1 teaspoon dried oregano

Salt and pepper to taste.

Preparation:

Cut the courgettes into julienne strips to obtain courgette "spaghetti". In a pan, heat the olive oil and add the onion and garlic. Fry until golden. Add the ground beef to the pan and cook until well browned. Add the tomato puree, oregano, salt and pepper. Mix well and cook over medium-low heat for about 15-20 minutes. Meanwhile, in another pan, cook the courgette "spaghetti" for 2-3 minutes until tender. Serve the courgette spaghetti with the ragù on top. Enjoy your meal!

FISH AND SEAFOOD SOUP

Preparation time: 15 minutes

Cooking times: 30 minutes

Ingredients:

Serves 4 people

500 g of mixed fish (cod ,

prawns, mussels, clams)

1 onion, chopped

2 cloves garlic, minced

400 g peeled tomatoes, chopped

1 liter of fish broth or water

1 teaspoon dried oregano

1 teaspoon red pepper flakes

Juice of 1 lemon

Chopped fresh parsley to taste

Salt and pepper to taste.

Olive oil for cooking

Preparation:

In a large pot, heat a drizzle of olive oil and add the onion and garlic. Fry until golden. Add the mixed fish to the pot and cook for a few minutes, until lightly browned. Add the chopped peeled tomatoes, the fish broth (or water), the oregano, the chilli pepper (if you like), the lemon juice, the salt and the pepper. Mix well and bring to the boil. Reduce the heat and cook over medium-low heat for about 20 to 25 minutes, or until the fish is cooked through and the flavors blend. Before serving, sprinkle with chopped fresh parsley. Serve the fish and seafood soup piping hot . Enjoy your meal!

CHICKEN SALAD WITH TOMATOES AND FETA CHEESE

Preparation time: 20 minutes

Cooking times: 15 minutes

Ingredients:

Serves 4 people

2 chicken breasts, cooked and diced

200 g cherry tomatoes, halved

100g feta cheese, crumbled

1 cucumber, cut into thin slices

1 yellow pepper, diced

1 red onion, thinly sliced

Juice of 1 lemon

3 tablespoons of olive oil

Chopped fresh parsley to taste

Salt and pepper to taste.

Preparation:

In a large bowl, combine the chicken cubes, cherry tomatoes, feta cheese, cucumber, yellow bell pepper and red onion. In a separate small bowl, whisk together the lemon juice, olive oil, salt and pepper to make the sauce. Pour the dressing into the bowl of ingredients and mix well to dress the salad. Sprinkle with chopped fresh parsley to garnish. Serve the chicken salad with cherry tomatoes and feta. Enjoy your meal!

ZUCCHINI LINGUINE WITH TOMATO SAUCE AND GRILLED CHICKEN

Preparation time: 20 minutes

Cooking times: 30 minutes

Ingredients:

Serves 4 people

4 courgettes

2 chicken breasts marinated in olive oil ,

lemon juice, salt, pepper and spices to taste

400 g peeled tomatoes, chopped

1 onion, chopped, 2 cloves garlic, chopped

1 tablespoon olive oil

Salt and pepper to taste.

Chopped fresh basil to taste

Preparation:

Using a spiralizer or potato peeler, create courgette "linguine". Set them aside. In a pan, heat the olive oil and add the onion and garlic. Fry until golden. Add the peeled tomatoes cut into pieces, salt and pepper. Mix well and cook over medium-low heat for about 15-20 minutes. Meanwhile, grill the marinated chicken breasts until cooked through. Add the zucchini linguine to the tomato sauce and stir to evenly distribute the sauce. Serve zucchini linguine with tomato sauce and grilled chicken on top. Sprinkle with chopped fresh basil and grated cheese, if desired. Enjoy your meal!

CAULIFLOWER RISOTTO WITH MUSHROOMS AND GRATED CHEESE

Preparation time: 15 minutes

Cooking times: 25 minutes

Ingredients:

Serves 4 people

1 medium cauliflower, cut into small pieces

200g mixed mushrooms, cut into slices

1 onion, chopped

2 cloves garlic, minced

300 g of Arborio or Carnaroli rice

1/2 glass of dry white wine

1 liter of vegetable broth

50 g of grated parmesan

2 tablespoons of olive oil

Salt and pepper to taste.

Preparation:

In a large pot, bring the vegetable broth to the boil and keep it warm. In a pan, heat the olive oil and add the onion and garlic. Fry until golden. Add the mushrooms to the pan and cook until golden brown and the released water has evaporated. Set them aside. In another pan, add the rice and toast it for a few minutes, stirring constantly. Add the white wine to the pan with the rice and mix until completely absorbed.

Add the cauliflower cut into pieces to the pan and begin adding the vegetable broth little by little, stirring constantly and waiting for the broth to absorb before adding more. Continue adding the broth and stirring until the rice is cooked al dente and the cauliflower is soft. Add the sautéed mushrooms to the pan with the risotto and mix well. Season with salt and pepper according to your taste. Before serving, sprinkle with grated cheese. Serve the cauliflower risotto with mushrooms and grated cheese hot. Enjoy your meal!

CHICKEN BROTH SOUP WITH VEGETABLES

Preparation time: 15 minutes

Cooking times: 30 minutes

Ingredients:

Serves 4 people

1 liter chicken broth (homemade or purchased)

2 chicken breasts, cooked and diced

2 carrots, cut into rounds

2 stalks celery, cut into slices

1 onion, chopped

2 cloves garlic, minced

100 g peas (fresh or frozen)

1 courgette, cut into cubes

Chopped fresh parsley to taste

Salt and pepper to taste. Olive oil for cooking

Preparation:

In a large pot, heat a drizzle of olive oil and add the onion and garlic. Fry until golden. Add the carrots, celery and courgette to the pot and cook for a few minutes, until slightly softened. Pour the chicken broth into the pot and bring to a boil. Reduce the heat and add the peas and cooked chicken cubes. Cook over medium-low heat for about 15-20 minutes, or until the vegetables are tender. Taste and adjust salt and pepper to your taste. Before serving, sprinkle with chopped fresh parsley. Serve the chicken broth soup with vegetables hot. Enjoy your meal!

TUNA SALAD WITH BOILED EGGS AND OLIVES

Preparation time: 15 minutes

Cooking times: 10 minutes

Ingredients:

Serves 4 people

2 cans of tuna in oil, drained

4 hard-boiled eggs, cut in half

200 g cherry tomatoes, halved

100 g of black olives, pitted and cut into slices

1 red onion, thinly sliced

Juice of 1 lemon

3 tablespoons of olive oil

Chopped fresh parsley to taste

Salt and pepper to taste.

Preparation:

In a large bowl, combine the drained tuna, the hard-boiled eggs cut in half, the cherry tomatoes, the olives and the red onion. In a separate small bowl, whisk together the lemon juice, olive oil, salt and pepper to make the sauce. Pour the dressing into the bowl of ingredients and mix well to dress the salad. Sprinkle with chopped fresh parsley to garnish. Serve the tuna salad with hard-boiled eggs and olives. Enjoy your meal!

CUCUMBER TAGLIATELLE WITH TUNA SAUCE AND TOMATOES

Preparation time: 15 minutes

Cooking times: none

Ingredients:

Serves 4 people

2 cucumbers

2 cans of drained tuna

200 g cherry tomatoes, halved

1 red onion, thinly sliced

Juice of 1 lemon, 3 tablespoons of olive oil

Chopped fresh parsley to taste

Salt and pepper to taste.

Preparation:

Using a vegetable peeler, create cucumber "noodles." Set them aside. In a bowl, combine the drained tuna, cherry tomatoes, red onion, lemon juice, olive oil, salt and pepper. Mix well to obtain the tuna sauce. Add the cucumber "noodles" to the bowl with the tuna sauce and toss gently to coat the noodles. Serve the cucumber tagliatelle with the tuna and cherry tomato sauce. Sprinkle with chopped fresh parsley. Enjoy your meal!

ZUCCHINI SPAGHETTI WITH SPINACH PESTO AND CHICKEN

Preparation time: 20 minutes

Cooking time: 15 minutes

Ingredient:

Serves 4 people

4 courgettes

200g chicken breast, cut into cubes

100 g of fresh spinach

30 g of walnuts

2 cloves of garlic

50 g grated Parmesan

Juice of 1/2 citron

3 tablespoons olive oil, Salt and pepper to taste.

Preparation:

Using a spiralizer or potato peeler, create zucchini "spaghetti". Set them aside. In a pan, heat a tablespoon of olive oil and cook the chicken cubes until cooked through and golden brown. Set it aside. In a blender or blender, combine spinach, walnuts, garlic, grated Parmesan, lemon juice, salt and pepper. Blend until you obtain a creamy consistency. Gradually add olive oil until desired consistency is achieved. In a pan, heat the courgette "spaghetti" with a spoonful of olive oil until tender. Add the spinach pesto to the pan with the courgette "spaghetti" and mix well to season the spaghetti. Add the cooked chicken to the skillet and stir gently. Serve the zucchini "spaghetti" with spinach and chicken pesto. Enjoy your meal!

VEGETABLE SOUP WITH TURKEY MEATBALLS

Preparation time: 20 minutes

Cooking times: 30 minutes

Ingredients:

Serves 4 people

500 g of minced turkey meat

1 onion, chopped, 2 carrots, diced

2 stalks celery, diced

1 courgette, diced

2 cloves garlic, minced

1 liter of vegetable broth

2 tablespoons of olive oil

Chopped fresh parsley to taste

Salt and pepper to taste.

Preparation:

In a bowl, mix the ground turkey, chopped onion, chopped garlic, chopped fresh parsley, salt and pepper. Form meatballs of the desired size. In a saucepan, heat the olive oil and fry the onion and garlic until golden brown. Add the carrots, celery and courgette to the pot and cook for a few minutes, until slightly softened. Pour the vegetable broth into the pan and bring to the boil. Reduce the heat and add the turkey meatballs to the pot. Cook over medium-low heat for about 15 to 20 minutes, or until the meatballs are cooked through and the vegetables are tender. Taste and adjust salt and pepper to your taste. Before serving, sprinkle with chopped fresh parsley. Serve the vegetable soup with the turkey meatballs piping hot.

COURGETTE PAD THAI WITH PRAWNS

Preparation time: 20 minutes

Cooking times: 10 minutes

Ingredients:, Serves 4 people

4 courgettes, cut into julienne or spirals

200 g of peeled prawns

2 beaten eggs, Juice of 1 lemon

3 tablespoons soy sauce

2 tablespoons of brown sugar

3 tablespoons sesame oil

4 cloves of garlic minced

Preparation:

In a pan, heat the sesame oil and chopped garlic. Fry until the garlic is golden.

Add the shrimp to the pan and cook until pink and cooked through. Remove the shrimp from the pan and set aside. Pour the beaten eggs into the same pan and cook them until they are slightly thickened. Add the julienned courgettes to the pan and cook for a few minutes, until tender but still crunchy. In a separate bowl, whisk together the soy sauce, brown sugar, and lemon juice. Pour the sauce into the pan with the courgettes and mix well. Add the previously cooked prawns to the pan and mix gently to evenly distribute the sauce. If you want a little heat, add chili flakes to the pan and mix well. Before serving, garnish with pieces of toasted peanuts and chopped fresh coriander. Serve the courgette Pad Thai with prawns piping hot. Enjoy your meal!

CHICKEN SALAD WITH AVOCADO AND DRIED TOMATOES

Preparation time: 20 minutes

Cooking time: 15 minutes (for chicken)

Ingredients:

Serves 4 people

2 chicken breasts marinated in olive oil ,

lemon juice, salt, pepper and spices to taste

2 avocados , diced, Juice of 1 lemon

100g dried tomatoes, soaked

hot water and cut into strips

200 g of mixed lettuce ,

washed and cut into pieces

1 red onion, thinly sliced

3 tablespoons of olive oil

Salt and pepper to taste.

Preparation:

Grill the marinated chicken breasts until cooked through. Let them cool and cut them into slices or cubes. In a large bowl, combine grilled chicken, diced avocados , diced sun-dried tomatoes, mixed lettuce, and sliced red onion. In a separate small bowl, whisk together the lemon juice, olive oil, salt and pepper to make the sauce. Pour the dressing into the bowl of ingredients and mix well to dress the salad. Serve the chicken salad with avocado and sun-dried tomatoes. Enjoy your meal!

CAULIFLOWER RICE WITH GRILLED CHICKEN AND VEGETABLES

Preparation time: 20 minutes

Cooking times: 15 minutes

Ingredients:

Serves 4 people

2 chicken breasts, marinated in oil

olive oil, lemon juice, salt, pepper

1 medium cauliflower, cut into small pieces

2 carrots, cut into cubes

1 courgette, cut into cubes

1 red pepper, diced

1 onion, chopped, 2 cloves garlic, chopped

2 tablespoons of olive oil

Salt and pepper to taste.

Preparation:

Grill the marinated chicken breasts until cooked through. Let them cool and cut them into slices or cubes. In a blender or mixer, blend the chopped cauliflower until it becomes a rice-like consistency. In a large skillet, heat the olive oil and add the onion and garlic. Fry until golden brown. Add the vegetables (carrots, courgettes, peppers) to the pan and cook for 5-7 minutes, until tender but still crunchy. Add the cauliflower rice to the pan with the vegetables and mix well to season the rice. Taste and adjust salt and pepper to your taste. Serve cauliflower rice with grilled chicken and vegetables. Enjoy your meal!

BROCCOLI CREAM SOUP WITH GRATED CHEESE

Preparation time: 15 minutes

Cooking times: 25 minutes

Ingredients:

Serves 4 people

500 g broccoli, cut into pieces

1 onion, chopped

2 cloves garlic, minced

1 liter of vegetable broth

100 g of grated parmesan

2 tablespoons of olive oil

Salt and pepper to taste.

Preparation:

In a large pot, heat the olive oil and add the onion and garlic. Fry until golden. Add the broccoli to the pot and cook for a few minutes, until slightly softened. Pour the vegetable broth into the pan and bring to the boil. Reduce heat and cook over medium-low heat for about 15 to 20 minutes, or until broccoli is tender. Using an immersion blender or blender, blend the soup until smooth and creamy. Taste and adjust salt and pepper to your taste. Before serving, sprinkle with grated cheese. Serve the broccoli cream with the grated cheese piping hot. Enjoy your meal!

ZUCCHINI SPAGHETTI WITH TOMATO SAUCE AND CHICKEN MEATBALLS

Preparation time: 30 minutes

Cooking times: 30 minutes

Ingredients:

Serves 4 people

4 courgettes

400 g peeled tomatoes, chopped

500 g of minced chicken meat

1 onion, chopped, 2 cloves garlic, chopped

1 egg, 50 g of breadcrumbs

Chopped fresh parsley to taste

Salt and pepper to taste.

Olive oil for cooking

Preparation:

Using a spiralizer or potato peeler, create zucchini "spaghetti". Set them aside. In a bowl, mix the minced chicken, chopped onion, chopped garlic, egg, breadcrumbs, chopped fresh parsley, salt and pepper. Form meatballs of the desired size. In a pan, heat a drizzle of olive oil and cook the chicken meatballs until cooked and golden. Set them aside. In a separate pan, heat a drizzle of olive oil and add the peeled tomatoes cut into pieces, salt and pepper. Cook over medium-low heat for about 15-20 minutes, or until the sauce has thickened.

Add the zucchini "spaghetti" to the pan with the tomato sauce and stir to evenly distribute the sauce. Add the chicken meatballs to the pan with the zucchini "spaghetti" and tomato sauce. Stir gently to combine the ingredients. Before serving, sprinkle with chopped fresh parsley. Serve the zucchini spaghetti with tomato sauce and chicken meatballs. Enjoy your meal!

TOMATO SOUP WITH BASIL AND CRISPY BACON

Preparation time: 15 minutes

Cooking times: 30 minutes

Ingredients:

Serves 4 people

1 kg of ripe tomatoes, cut into cubes

1 onion, chopped

2 cloves garlic, minced

4 slices of bacon, cut into strips

1 bunch fresh basil, chopped

2 tablespoons of olive oil

Salt and pepper to taste.

Preparation:

In a large pot, heat the olive oil and add the onion and garlic. Fry until golden. Add the diced tomatoes to the pot and cook over medium heat for about 20-25 minutes, until the tomatoes have softened and the sauce has thickened slightly. Meanwhile, in a separate skillet, cook bacon over medium-high heat until crisp. Set it aside. Add the chopped basil to the pan with the tomato puree and mix well. Blend the soup with an immersion blender or mixer until you obtain a smooth and homogeneous consistency. Taste and adjust salt and pepper to your taste. Before serving, garnish each portion with crispy bacon. Serve the tomato soup with basil and hot crispy bacon. Enjoy your meal!

TUNA SALAD WITH AVOCADO AND CUCUMBER

Preparation time: 15 minutes

Cooking times: 0 minutes

Ingredients:

Serves 4 people

2 cans of tuna in oil, drained

2 avocados , diced

2 cucumbers, cut into rounds

Juice of 1 lemon

2 tablespoons of olive oil

Chopped fresh parsley to taste

Salt and pepper to taste.

Preparation:

In a large bowl, combine the drained tuna, diced avocados , and diced cucumbers. In a separate small bowl, whisk together the lemon juice, olive oil, salt and pepper to make the sauce. Pour the dressing into the bowl of ingredients and mix well to dress the salad. Sprinkle with chopped fresh parsley to garnish. Serve tuna salad with avocado and cucumber. Enjoy your meal!

CUCUMBER NOODLES WITH TOMATO SAUCE AND SAUSAGE

Preparation time: 15 minutes

Cooking times: 30 minutes

Ingredients:

Serves 4 people

2 cucumbers

200 g of sausage, peeled and crumbled

400 g peeled tomatoes, chopped

1 onion, chopped, 2 cloves garlic, chopped

2 tablespoons of olive oil

1 teaspoon of sugar

Chopped fresh basil to taste

Salt and pepper to taste.

Preparation:

Using a spiralizer or vegetable peeler, create cucumber "noodles." Set them aside. In a pan, heat the olive oil and add the onion and garlic. Fry until golden. Add the crumbled sausage to the pan and cook until cooked through. Add the peeled tomatoes cut into pieces, salt, pepper and sugar to the pan. Mix well and cook over medium-low heat for about 15-20 minutes, or until the sauce has thickened. Add the cucumber "noodles" to the pan with the tomato sauce and stir to evenly distribute the sauce. Before serving, garnish with chopped fresh basil. Serve the cucumber tagliatelle with tomato sauce and sausage. Enjoy your meal!

CAULIFLOWER RISOTTO WITH SHRIMP AND GRATED CHEESE

Preparation time: 20 minutes

Cooking times: 30 minutes

Ingredients:

Serves 4 people

1 medium cauliflower ,

cut into small pieces

300 g of peeled prawns

1 onion, chopped, 2 cloves garlic, chopped

300 g of Arborio rice

1/2 glass of dry white wine

1 liter of vegetable broth

50 g of grated parmesan

2 tablespoons of olive oil

Chopped fresh parsley to taste

Salt and pepper to taste.

Preparation:

Bring the vegetable broth to the boil in a saucepan and keep warm over low heat. In another pot, heat the olive oil and add the onion and garlic. Fry until golden. Add the Arborio rice to the pan and toast it for a few minutes, stirring constantly. Deglaze with dry white wine and let the alcohol evaporate. Add the hot vegetable broth little by little, one ladle at a time, stirring constantly and waiting for the broth to absorb before adding the next one.

Add the cauliflower pieces to the pot about halfway through cooking the risotto and continue cooking until the rice and cauliflower are tender. Add the peeled prawns to the pot and stir well to distribute the ingredients. Taste and adjust salt and pepper to your taste. Before serving, sprinkle with grated cheese and chopped fresh parsley. Serve the cauliflower risotto with prawns and grated cheese. Enjoy your meal!

MUSHROOM SOUP WITH CREAM AND PARSLEY

Preparation time: 15 minutes

Cooking times: 25 minutes

Ingredients:

Serves 4 people

500 g of mixed mushrooms ,

cleaned and sliced, 1 onion, chopped

2 cloves garlic, minced

500 ml of vegetable broth

200 ml of cooking cream

2 tablespoons of olive oil

Chopped fresh parsley to taste

Salt and pepper to taste.

Preparation:

In a large pot, heat the olive oil and add the onion and garlic. Fry until golden. Add the sliced mushrooms to the pot and cook until soft and golden. Pour the vegetable broth into the pan and bring to the boil. Lower the heat and simmer over medium-low heat for about 15-20 minutes. Using an immersion blender or blender, partially blend the soup to a slightly creamy consistency. Add the cooking cream to the pan and mix well. Taste and adjust salt and pepper to your taste. Before serving, garnish with chopped fresh parsley. Serve the mushroom soup with cream and parsley piping hot . Enjoy your meal!

CHICKEN SALAD WITH GRILLED VEGETABLES AND FETA CHEESE

Preparation time: 20 minutes

Cooking times: 15 minutes

Ingredients:

Serves 4 people

2 chicken breasts marinated in olive oil ,

lemon juice, salt, pepper and spices to taste

2 courgettes, cut into thin slices

1 yellow pepper, cut into strips

1 red pepper, cut into strips

1 red onion, thinly sliced

200 g of mixed lettuce, washed and cut into pieces

100g feta cheese, crumbled

3 tablespoons of olive oil, juice of 1 lemon

Chopped fresh parsley to taste

Salt and pepper to taste.

Preparation:

Grill the marinated chicken breasts until cooked through. Let them cool and cut them into slices or cubes. In a grill or grill pan, grill the zucchini slices, yellow and red bell pepper strips, and onion slices until tender and lightly smoky. In a large bowl, combine the grilled chicken, grilled vegetables, lettuce and crumbled feta cheese. In a separate small bowl, whisk together the olive oil, lemon juice, salt and pepper to make the sauce. Pour the dressing into the bowl of ingredients and mix well to dress the salad. Sprinkle with chopped fresh parsley to garnish. Serve the chicken salad with grilled vegetables and feta cheese.

ZUCCHINI LINGUINE WITH TOMATO SAUCE AND OVEN COOKED CHICKEN

Preparation time: 20 minutes

Cooking times: 30 minutes

Ingredients:

Serves 4 people

4 courgettes, cut into linguine with

a spiralizer or potato peeler

400g chicken breast, cut into cubes

400 g peeled tomatoes, chopped

1 onion, chopped

2 cloves garlic, minced

2 tablespoons of olive oil

1 teaspoon of sugar

Chopped fresh basil to taste

Salt and pepper to taste.

Preparation:

In a pan, heat the olive oil and add the onion and garlic. Fry until golden. Add the cubed chicken to the pan and cook until cooked through. Add the peeled tomatoes cut into pieces, salt, pepper and sugar to the pan. Mix well and cook over medium-low heat for about 15-20 minutes, or until the sauce has thickened. Add the zucchini linguine to the pan with the tomato sauce and stir to evenly distribute the sauce. Before serving, garnish with chopped fresh basil. Serve the courgette linguine with tomato sauce and baked chicken. Enjoy your meal!

TOMATO SOUP WITH

SHRIMP AND BASIL

Preparation time: 15 minutes

Cooking times: 25 minutes

Ingredients:

Serves 4 people

400 g of peeled prawns

800 g peeled tomatoes, chopped

1 onion, chopped

2 cloves garlic, minced

2 tablespoons of olive oil

1 teaspoon of sugar

1 bunch fresh basil, chopped

Salt and pepper to taste.

Preparation:

In a large pot, heat the olive oil and add the onion and garlic. Fry until golden. Add the peeled tomatoes cut into pieces, salt, pepper and sugar to the pan. Mix well and cook over medium-low heat for about 15-20 minutes, or until the sauce has thickened. Using an immersion blender or blender, partially blend the soup until it has a consistency with tomato chunks. Add the peeled prawns to the pan and cook for a few minutes, until well cooked. Add the chopped basil to the pot and mix well. Taste and adjust salt and pepper to your taste. Before serving, garnish with fresh basil leaves. Serve the tomato soup with prawns and basil piping hot .

TUNA SALAD WITH BOILED EGGS AND AVOCADO

Preparation time: 15 minutes

Cooking times: 10 minutes

Ingredients:

Serves 4 people

2 cans of tuna in oil, drained

4 eggs, hard-boiled and sliced

2 avocados , diced

200 g of mixed lettuce ,

washed and torn to pieces

1 red onion, thinly sliced

Juice of 1 lemon, 3 tablespoons of olive oil

Salt and pepper to taste.

Preparation:

In a large bowl, combine the drained tuna, sliced hard-boiled eggs, diced avocados, sautéed lettuce and sliced red onion . In a separate small bowl, whisk together the lemon juice, olive oil, salt and pepper to make the sauce. Pour the dressing into the bowl of ingredients and mix well to dress the salad. Serve the tuna salad with hard-boiled eggs and avocado. Enjoy your meal!

CUCUMBER TAGLIOLINI WITH TUNA SAUCE AND DRIED TOMATOES

Preparation time: 15 minutes

Cooking times: none

Ingredients:

Serves 4, 2 cucumbers

2 cans of tuna in oil, drained

100g dried tomatoes, soaked

hot water and cut into strips

Juice of 1 lemon

3 tablespoons of olive oil

Chopped fresh parsley to taste

Salt and pepper to taste.

Preparation:

Using a spiralizer or vegetable peeler, create cucumber "noodles." Set them aside. In a large bowl, combine the drained tuna, the dried tomatoes cut into strips, the lemon juice, the olive oil, the salt and the pepper. Mix the tuna sauce well until you obtain a homogeneous mixture. Add the cucumber "noodles" to the bowl with the tuna sauce and mix gently to evenly distribute the sauce. Before serving, sprinkle with chopped fresh parsley. Serve the cucumber tagliatelle with tuna sauce and dried tomatoes. Enjoy your meal!

CAULIFLOWER RICE WITH GRILLED CHICKEN AND SPINACH

Preparation time: 20 minutes

Cooking times: 25 minutes

Ingredients:

Serves 4 people

1 medium cauliflower, cut into small pieces

400 g chicken breast marinated in olive oil ,

lemon juice, salt, pepper and spices to taste

200 g of fresh spinach

1 onion, chopped

2 cloves garlic, minced

2 tablespoons of olive oil

Salt and pepper to taste.

Preparation:

In a food processor, blend the cauliflower until it resembles rice. In a pan, heat the olive oil and add the onion and garlic. Fry until golden. Add the chopped cauliflower to the pan and cook for a few minutes until tender. Meanwhile, grill the marinated chicken breast until cooked through. Let it cool and cut it into slices or cubes. Add the fresh spinach to the pan with the cauliflower and stir until the spinach is wilted. Season with salt and pepper according to your taste. Before serving, add the chicken slices or cubes to the pan and stir gently to combine the ingredients. Serve cauliflower rice with grilled chicken and spinach. Enjoy your meal!

VEGETABLE SOUP WITH TURKEY MEATBALLS AND LEMON

Preparation time: 20 minutes

Cooking times: 30 minutes

Ingredients:

Serves 4 people

500 g of minced turkey meat

Juice and grated zest of 1 lemon

1 egg, 50 g of breadcrumbs

Chopped fresh parsley to taste

Salt and pepper to taste.

1 liter of vegetable broth

2 carrots, cut into rounds, 2 courgettes, cut

1 onion, chopped, 2 cloves garlic, chopped

2 tablespoons olive oil, Salt and pepper to taste.

Preparation:

In a bowl, mix the ground turkey meat, grated lemon zest, juice, egg, breadcrumbs, chopped fresh parsley, salt and pepper. Form meatballs of the desired size. In a saucepan, heat the olive oil and add the onion and garlic. Fry until golden. Add the carrots and zucchini to the pot and cook until tender. Pour the vegetable broth into the pan and bring to the boil. Reduce the heat and add the turkey meatballs to the pot. Cook over medium-low heat for about 15-20 minutes, or until the meatballs are cooked through. Taste and adjust salt and pepper to your taste. Before serving, sprinkle with chopped fresh parsley. Serve the vegetable soup with the hot lemon turkey meatballs . Enjoy your meal!

ZUCCHINI PAD THAI WITH CHICKEN AND PEANUT SAUCE

Preparation time: 20 minutes

Cooking times: 15 minutes

Ingredients:

Serves 4 people

2 courgettes, cut into

julienne or spirals

400g chicken breast, cut into strips

200 g of soya sprouts

3 tablespoons soy sauce

2 tablespoons fish sauce

2 tablespoons of brown sugar

1 tablespoon rice vinegar

Juice of 1 lemon

3 tablespoons peanut sauce

2 tablespoons peanut oil

Fresh spring onion, cut into thin rings

Toasted cashews, chopped to taste

Preparation:

In a bowl, mix the soy sauce, fish sauce, brown sugar, rice vinegar, lemon juice and peanut sauce to make the sauce. In a skillet or wok, heat the peanut oil over medium-high heat. Add the chicken and cook until browned and cooked through. Add the julienned courgettes and bean sprouts to the pan and cook for a few minutes until tender.

Pour the prepared sauce into the pan and mix well to season the ingredients. Also, add crushed red pepper if you prefer a spicy touch. Continue stirring until all the ingredients are well combined and the sauce has coated the zucchini and chicken. Before serving, garnish with thinly sliced fresh onion and chopped cashews. Serve the zucchini pad Thai with chicken and peanut sauce. Enjoy your meal!

CHICKEN SALAD WITH AVOCADO DRIED TOMATOES AND FETA CHEESE

Preparation time: 15 minutes

Cooking times: none

Ingredients:

Serves 4 people

400 g of chicken breast cooked and cut into strips

2 avocados , diced

100g dried tomatoes, soaked

hot water and cut into small pieces

100g feta cheese, crumbled

200 g of mixed lettuce, washed and cut into pieces

1 red onion, thinly sliced

Juice of 1 lemon

3 tablespoons of olive oil, Salt and pepper to taste.

Preparation:

In a large bowl, combine cooked chicken strips, diced avocados , diced sun-dried tomatoes, mixed lettuce, and sliced red onion. In a separate small bowl, whisk together the lemon juice, olive oil, salt and pepper to make the sauce. Pour the dressing into the bowl of ingredients and mix well to dress the salad. Add the crumbled feta to the bowl and mix gently to evenly distribute the cheese. Serve the chicken salad with avocado, sun-dried tomatoes and feta cheese. Enjoy your meal!

CAULIFLOWER RISOTTO WITH CRISPY BACON AND GRATED CHEESE

Preparation time: 15 minutes

Cooking times: 25 minutes

Ingredients:

Serves 4 people

1 medium cauliflower, cut into small pieces

200g bacon, cut into cubes

1 onion, chopped, 2 cloves of garlic

300 g of Arborio or Carnaroli rice

1/2 glass of dry white wine

1.2 liters vegetable broth, boiling

50 g of grated parmesan

2 tablespoons butter, Salt and pepper to taste.

Preparation:

In a food processor, blend the cauliflower until it resembles rice. In a large saucepan, brown the bacon until crispy. Remove the bacon from the pan and set aside. In the same pot, add the onion and garlic and fry until golden brown. Add the rice to the pan and toast it for about 2 minutes, stirring constantly. Add the white wine and let it evaporate. Add the hot vegetable broth little by little, one ladle at a time, stirring constantly and waiting for the broth to absorb before adding the next one. After about 15-20 minutes of cooking , add the chopped cauliflower and continue to cook until the rice is al dente and the cauliflower is tender. Remove the pan from the heat and add the grated cheese and butter. Mix well until the cheese and butter have melted into the risotto. Taste and adjust salt and pepper to your taste. Before serving, garnish with crispy bacon. Serve the cauliflower risotto with crispy bacon and grated cheese. Enjoy your meal!

TOMATO SOUP WITH SHRIMP AND BASIL

Preparation time: 15 minutes

Cooking times: 25 minutes

Ingredients:

Serves 4 people

400 g of peeled prawns

800 g peeled tomatoes, chopped

1 onion, chopped

2 cloves garlic, minced

2 tablespoons of olive oil

1 teaspoon of sugar

1 bunch fresh basil, chopped

Salt and pepper to taste.

Preparation:

In a large pot, heat the olive oil and add the onion and garlic. Fry until golden. Add the peeled tomatoes cut into pieces, salt, pepper and sugar to the pan. Mix well and cook over medium-low heat for about 15-20 minutes, or until the sauce has thickened. Using an immersion blender or blender, partially blend the soup until it has a consistency with tomato chunks. Add the peeled prawns to the pan and cook for a few minutes, until well cooked. Add the chopped basil to the pot and mix well. Taste and adjust salt and pepper to your taste. Before serving, garnish with fresh basil leaves. Serve the tomato soup with prawns and basil piping hot . Enjoy your meal!

TUNA SALAD WITH AVOCADO, CUCUMBERS , AND BLACK OLIVES

Preparation time: 15 minutes

Cooking times: none

Ingredients:

Serves 4 people

2 cans of tuna in oil, drained

2 avocados , diced

2 cucumbers, cut into rounds

100 g of black olives, pitted and sliced

Juice of 1 lemon

3 tablespoons of olive oil

Salt and pepper to taste.

Preparation:

In a large bowl, combine the drained tuna, diced avocados , diced cucumbers and sliced black olives. In a separate small bowl, whisk together the lemon juice, olive oil, salt and pepper to make the sauce. Pour the dressing into the bowl of ingredients and mix well to dress the salad. Serve the tuna salad with avocado, cucumber and black olives. Enjoy your meal!

CUCUMBER NOODLES WITH TOMATO SAUCE AND BAKED SAUSAGE

Preparation time: 20 minutes

Cooking times: 30 minutes

Ingredients:

Serves 4 people

2 cucumbers

400g sausage, skinned and crumbled

400 g peeled tomatoes, chopped

1 onion, chopped

2 cloves garlic, minced

2 tablespoons of olive oil

1 teaspoon of sugar

Chopped fresh basil, Salt and pepper to taste.

Preparation:

Using a spiralizer or vegetable peeler, create cucumber "noodles." Set them aside. In a pan, heat the olive oil and add the onion and garlic. Fry until golden. Add the crumbled sausage to the pan and cook until cooked through. Add the peeled tomatoes cut into pieces, salt, pepper and sugar to the pan. Mix well and cook over medium-low heat for about 15-20 minutes, or until the sauce has thickened. Add the cucumber "tagliatelle" to the pan with the tomato and sausage sauce. Stir to evenly distribute the sauce. Before serving, garnish with chopped fresh basil. Serve cucumber tagliatelle with tomato sauce and baked sausage. Enjoy your meal!

RECIPES
SECOND DISHES

GRILLED CHICKEN WITH AVOCADO SAUCE

Preparation time: 15 minutes

Cooking time: 10-15 minutes

Doses for: 4 people

Ingredients:

4 skinless, boneless chicken breasts

Salt and pepper to taste

1 ripe avocado, mashed

60 ml fresh lime juice

30 g chopped fresh coriander

1 clove garlic, minced

1/4 teaspoon cumin powder

1/4 teaspoon chili powder

1/8 teaspoon salt

Preparation:

Preheat grill to medium-high heat. Season the chicken with salt and pepper. In a bowl, mix the avocado, lime juice, cilantro, garlic, cumin, chili powder and salt. Grill chicken for 5-7 minutes per side, or until cooked through. Serve the chicken with the avocado sauce on top.

GRILLED BEEF STEAK WITH GRILLED VEGETABLES

Preparation time: 10 minutes

(marinating) + 10 minutes

Cooking times: 15-20 minutes

Ingredients:

Serves 4 people

4 beef steaks, preferably

cuts such as sirloin or T-Bone steak, 2 zucchini, cut into long slices

1 aubergine, cut into long slices

1 red pepper, cut into strips

1 yellow pepper, cut into strips

2 tablespoons of olive oil

Juice of 1 lemon, 2 cloves of garlic, chopped

Salt and pepper to taste.

Preparation:

Marinate the beef steaks in lemon juice, minced garlic, salt, pepper and olive oil for at least 10 minutes. Heat a grill or skillet over medium-high heat. Grill beef steaks for 5-7 minutes per side or until desired doneness. Let the steaks rest for a few minutes before slicing. Meanwhile, in the same grill or skillet, grill the zucchini, eggplant, and peppers until tender and lightly smoky. Brush the vegetables with olive oil while cooking. Season with salt and pepper. Slice the beef steaks and serve with the grilled vegetables as a side dish. Serve the grilled beef steak with a side of grilled vegetables. Enjoy your meal!

CHICKEN BREAST WITH LEMON WITH SAUTEED SPINACH

Preparation time: 10 minutes (marinating) + 15 minutes

Cooking times: 15-20 minutes

Ingredients:

Serves 4 people

4 chicken breasts, skinless and boneless

Juice and grated zest of 2 lemons

2 tablespoons of olive oil

2 cloves garlic, minced

200 g of fresh spinach

Salt and pepper to taste.

Preparation:

Marinate the chicken breasts in lemon juice, grated lemon zest, minced garlic, salt, pepper and olive oil for at least 10 minutes. Heat a skillet over medium-high heat and add the marinated chicken breasts. Cook for 6-8 minutes per side, or until cooked through and golden brown. While the chicken is cooking, heat a separate pan with a little olive oil. Add the chopped garlic and fry for a few seconds. Add fresh spinach to the pan and sauté until wilted and reduced in volume. Squeeze the juice of 1 lemon over the sautéed spinach. Season with salt and pepper. Serve the lemon chicken breasts on a bed of sautéed spinach. Serve the lemon chicken breast with sautéed spinach. Enjoy your meal!

GRILLED SALMON WITH AVOCADO SAUCE

Preparation time: 20 minutes

Cooking times: 10-15 minutes

Ingredients:

Serves 4 people

4 salmon fillets, skinless

2 ripe avocados , peeled and pitted

Juice of 1 lemon

2 tablespoons of olive oil

2 cloves garlic, minced

Salt and pepper to taste.

Preparation:

Marinate the salmon fillets in lemon juice, minced garlic, salt, pepper and olive oil for at least 10 minutes. Heat a grill or skillet over medium-high heat. Grill salmon fillets for 5-6 minutes per side, or until desired doneness. Meanwhile, in a blender or food processor, blend the avocados with lemon juice, minced garlic, salt and pepper until smooth. Serve the grilled salmon fillets with a generous spoonful of avocado sauce on top. Serve the grilled salmon with avocado salsa. Enjoy your meal!

BAKED TURKEY MEATBALLS WITH MIXED SALAD

Preparation time: 15 minutes

Cooking times: 25-30 minutes

Ingredients:

Serves 4 people

500 g of minced turkey meat

1 egg, 1/2 cup breadcrumbs

2 tablespoons grated cheese

2 cloves garlic, minced

Chopped fresh parsley to taste

Salt and pepper to taste. For the mixed salad:

Mixed salad, washed and cut into pieces

Cherry tomatoes, halved

Black olives, pitted, Olive oil dressing, Preparation:

In a bowl, combine the ground turkey, egg, breadcrumbs, grated cheese, minced garlic, parsley, salt and pepper. Mix well to combine the ingredients. Take small portions of dough and form meatballs of the desired size. Place the meatballs on a baking tray lined with baking paper. Cook the turkey meatballs in a preheated oven at 180°C for 25-30 minutes, or until cooked and golden. In the meantime, prepare the mixed salad by combining the lettuce, cherry tomatoes and black olives in a bowl. Season with olive oil , balsamic vinegar or dressing of your choice. Serve the baked turkey meatballs with the mixed salad as a side dish. Serve the baked turkey meatballs with a mixed salad.

PORK CHOPS WITH MUSHROOM SAUCE AND STEAMED BROCCOLI

Preparation time: 45 minutes

Cooking times: 30 minutes

Ingredients:

Serves 4 people

4 pork chops

200 g of mixed mushrooms

sliced, 1 onion, chopped

2 cloves garlic, minced

200 ml of meat broth

100 ml of cooking cream

2 tablespoons of olive oil

Chopped fresh parsley to taste

Salt and pepper to taste. For the side dish:

1 bunch broccoli, separated into florets

Juice of 1 lemon, salt to taste

Preparation:

Heat the olive oil in a skillet and brown the pork chops on both sides until golden brown. Remove them from the pan and set them aside. In the same pan, add the onion and garlic and fry until golden brown. Add the mushrooms to the pan and cook until tender. Add the beef broth and cooking cream to the pan. Bring to the boil and then reduce the heat. Let the sauce cook until it thickens slightly. Season with salt and pepper according to your taste.

Add the chopped fresh parsley and mix well. Return the pork chops to the skillet and cook over medium-low heat for another 10 to 15 minutes, until cooked through. Meanwhile, steam the broccoli until tender. Drain and season with lemon juice and salt. Serve the pork chops with the mushroom sauce, accompanied by steamed broccoli as a side dish. Enjoy your meal!

ROAST CHICKEN WITH SALAD OF ARUGULA AND TOMATOES

Preparation time: 15 minutes

Cooking times: 1 hour

Ingredients:

Serves 4 people

1 whole chicken, cleaned and dried

2 tablespoons of olive oil

2 cloves of garlic, minced, Juice of 1 lemon

1 teaspoon sweet paprika

Salt and pepper to taste.

For the arugula and cherry tomatoes:

200 g of rocket

200 g cherry tomatoes, halved

2 tablespoons balsamic vinegar

2 tablespoons olive oil, Salt and pepper to taste.

Preparation:

Preheat the oven to 180°C. In a bowl, mix olive oil, minced garlic, lemon juice, paprika, salt and pepper to create a marinade. Spread the marinade all over the chicken, making sure it is well covered. Transfer the chicken to a baking sheet and cook in the preheated oven for about 1 hour, or until the chicken is golden brown and cooked through. Meanwhile, in a large bowl, combine the arugula and cherry tomatoes. Season with balsamic vinegar, olive oil, salt and pepper. Mix well to distribute the seasoning. Once the chicken is cooked, let it rest for a few minutes, then slice it. Serve the roast chicken with the arugula and cherry tomato salad as a side dish. Enjoy your meal!

SOLE IN PIECE WITH STEAMED VEGETABLES

Preparation time: 15 minutes

Cooking times: 20 minutes

Ingredients:

Serves 4 people

4 sole fillets

1 courgette, thinly sliced

1 carrot, thinly sliced

1 onion, thinly sliced

Juice of 1 lemon

2 tablespoons of olive oil

Salt and pepper to taste.

Preparation:

Prepare four sheets of baking paper and place a fillet of sole on each. Distribute the slices of courgette, carrot and onion on each sole fillet. Season with lemon juice, olive oil, salt and pepper. Close the parcels carefully, folding the edges and sealing them well. Place the parcels on a baking tray and cook in a preheated oven at 180°C for about 20 minutes, or in any case until the fish is well cooked and the vegetables are tender. Serve the sole in foil with the steamed vegetables. Enjoy your meal!

GRILLED PRAWN SKEWERS WITH SAUTEED COURGETTES

Preparation time: 15 minutes

Cooking times: 10 minutes

Ingredients:

Serves 4 people

16-20 fresh prawns ,

peeled and peeled

2 courgettes, cut into thick rounds

Juice of 1 lemon

2 tablespoons of olive oil

Salt and pepper to taste.

Wooden skewers, previously

soaked in water

Preparation:

In a bowl, marinate the prawns with lemon juice, olive oil, salt and pepper for about 10 minutes. Thread the prawns on wooden skewers alternating them with slices of courgettes. Heat a grill or skillet over medium-high heat. Cook the shrimp skewers on the grill for about 2 to 3 minutes per side, or until the shrimp are pink and cooked through. Meanwhile, in a separate pan, heat a drizzle of olive oil and sauté the courgette slices until tender. Season the sautéed courgettes with salt and pepper to your taste. Serve the grilled shrimp skewers with the sautéed courgettes as a side dish. Enjoy your meal!

PORK FILLET WITH MUSTARD SAUCE AND BAKED CAULIFLOWER

Preparation time: 15 minutes

Cooking times: 30-40 minutes

Ingredients:

Serves 4, 4 pork fillets

2 tablespoons Dijon mustard

2 tablespoons honey

2 tablespoons of olive oil

2 cloves garlic, minced

Juice of 1 lemon

Salt and pepper to taste.

For the baked cauliflower side dish:

1 cauliflower, divided into florets

2 tablespoons of olive oil

2 cloves of garlic, minced, Salt and pepper to taste.

Preparation: Preheat the oven to 200°C. In a bowl, whisk together the Dijon mustard, honey, olive oil, minced garlic, lemon juice, salt, and pepper. Spread the sauce over the surface of the pork fillets. Transfer the pork tenderloins to a baking sheet and bake in the preheated oven for about 25 to 30 minutes, or until the pork is cooked through and browned. Meanwhile, in a bowl, toss the cauliflower florets with olive oil, minced garlic, salt and pepper. Place the seasoned cauliflower on a baking tray and bake in the preheated oven for approximately 20-25 minutes, or until the cauliflower is tender and lightly browned. Serve the pork fillet with mustard accompanied by the baked cauliflower as a side dish. Enjoy your meal!

CHICKEN CACCIATORA WITH ROASTED PEPPERS

Preparation time: 15 minutes

Cooking times: 40-50 minutes

Ingredients:

Serves 4 people

4 chicken thighs

1 onion, sliced,

2 cloves garlic, minced

400 g peeled tomatoes, chopped

200ml chicken broth

1 teaspoon dried oregano

1 teaspoon dried rosemary

1 teaspoon sweet paprika

Salt and pepper to taste.

For the roasted pepper side dish:

2 peppers (red and yellow), cut into strips

2 tablespoons olive oil,

Salt and pepper to taste.

Preparation:

Preheat the oven to 180°C. In a saucepan, heat a drizzle of olive oil and brown the chicken legs on both sides. Remove them from the pan and set them aside. In the same pot, add the onion and garlic and fry until golden brown. Add chopped canned tomatoes, chicken broth, oregano, rosemary, paprika, salt and pepper. Mix well. Return the chicken thighs to the pot with the tomato sauce.

Cover the pot and simmer over medium-low heat for about 30 to 40 minutes, or until the chicken is tender and cooked through. In the meantime, arrange the strips of peppers seasoned with oil, salt and pepper in a baking dish. Bake in the preheated oven for about 20-25 minutes, or until the peppers are soft and lightly caramelized. Serve the chicken Cacciatore with roasted peppers on the side. Enjoy your meal!

GRILLED TUNA WITH LIME SAUCE AND CUCUMBER SALAD

Preparation time: 15 minutes

Cooking times: 10 minutes

Ingredients:

Serves 4 people, 4 slices of fresh tuna

Juice and grated zest of 2 limes

2 tablespoons of olive oil

2 cloves garlic, minced

Salt and pepper to taste.

For the cucumber salad:

2 cucumbers, cut into thin rounds

2 tablespoons rice vinegar

1 teaspoon sugar, 1/2 teaspoon salt

Preparation:

In a bowl, mix together the lime juice, grated lime zest, olive oil, minced garlic, salt and pepper to create a marinade. Distribute the marinade over the tuna slices, taking care to cover them evenly. Heat a grill or skillet over medium-high heat. Grill the tuna slices for about 2 to 3 minutes per side, or until seared on the outside but still pink on the inside. Meanwhile, in a bowl, mix the ingredients for the cucumber salad: cucumbers, rice vinegar, sugar and salt. Mix well to combine the ingredients. Serve the grilled tuna with a generous dollop of the lime dressing and the cucumber salad on the side. Optionally, sprinkle the tuna slices with toasted sesame seeds for a crunchy touch. Enjoy your meal!

LAMB CHOPS WITH GRILLED ASPARAGUS

Preparation time: 15 minutes

Cooking times: 15-20 minutes

Ingredients:

Serves 4 people

8 lamb chops, 2 tablespoons olive oil

2 cloves garlic, minced

1 teaspoon dried rosemary

Salt and pepper to taste.

For the grilled asparagus side dish:

1 bunch of asparagus ,

slightly peeled bottoms

2 tablespoons of olive oil

Salt and pepper to taste.

Preparation:

Preheat grill or nonstick skillet over medium-high heat. In a bowl mix the olive oil, chopped garlic, rosemary, salt and pepper. Spread the marinade over the lamb chops, making sure they are evenly coated. Cook the lamb chops on the grill or pan for about 4-5 minutes per side, or until cooked to the desired degree. Meanwhile, in a bowl, season the asparagus with olive oil, salt and pepper. Grill the asparagus on the grill or in a pan for about 5-7 minutes, turning occasionally, or until tender and lightly caramelized. Serve the lamb chops with grilled asparagus on the side. Enjoy your meal!

CURRY CHICKEN WITH BAKED CAULIFLOWER

Preparation time: 15 minutes

Cooking times: 40 minutes

Ingredients:

Serves 4 people

4 chicken breasts, cut into cubes

1 cauliflower, divided into florets

1 onion, chopped

2 cloves garlic, minced

2 tablespoons curry powder

1 can coconut milk

2 tablespoons of olive oil

Salt and pepper to taste.

Preparation:

Preheat the oven to 200°C. In a pan, heat the olive oil and fry the onion and garlic until golden brown. Add the chicken to the pan and brown on all sides until browned. Add the curry powder and mix well to evenly coat the chicken. Add the cauliflower florets and coconut milk to the pan. Mix well to combine the ingredients. Transfer the pan to the preheated oven and cook for about 30 to 35 minutes, or until the chicken is cooked through and the cauliflower is tender. Taste and adjust salt and pepper to your taste. Serve the chicken curry with the baked cauliflower. Enjoy your meal!

BAKED SALMON WITH AVOCADO SAUCE AND SPINACH SALAD

Preparation time: 15 minutes

Cooking times: 15-20 minutes

Ingredients:

Serves 4 people

4 salmon fillets

2 ripe avocados , peeled and pitted

Juice of 1 lemon,

2 tablespoons of olive oil

2 cloves garlic, minced

Salt and pepper to taste.

For the spinach salad:

200 g of fresh spinach

200 g cherry tomatoes, halved

2 tablespoons balsamic vinegar

2 tablespoons olive oil, Salt and pepper to taste.

Preparation:

Preheat the oven to 200°C. In a bowl, mash the avocados and add the lemon juice, olive oil, minced garlic, salt and pepper. Mix well to obtain a smooth sauce. Place the salmon fillets on a baking tray lined with baking paper. Spread the avocado sauce over the salmon fillets. Bake the salmon in the preheated oven for about 12 to 15 minutes, or until the salmon is cooked to your liking. Meanwhile, in a large bowl, combine the spinach and cherry tomatoes. Season with balsamic vinegar, olive oil, salt and pepper. Mix well to distribute the seasoning. Serve the baked salmon with the avocado sauce accompanied by the spinach salad. Enjoy your meal!

BAKED BEEF MEATBALLS WITH GRATINUM COURGETTES

Preparation time: 15 minutes

Cooking times: 25-30 minutes

Ingredients:

Serves 4 people

500 g of minced meat, 1 egg

1/4 cup breadcrumbs

2 tablespoons chopped fresh parsley

1 clove garlic, minced

Salt and pepper to taste.

For the grated courgette side dish:

4 courgettes, cut into thin rounds

1/2 cup grated cheese

(e.g. parmesan or pecorino)

2 tablespoons of breadcrumbs

2 tablespoons of olive oil

Salt and pepper to taste.

Preparation:

Preheat the oven to 200°C. In a bowl, mix together the minced meat, egg, breadcrumbs, chopped parsley, chopped garlic, salt and pepper. Mix well to combine the ingredients. Form meatballs with the meat mixture and place them on a baking tray lined with baking paper. Place the meatballs in the preheated oven and bake for about 20-25 minutes, or until the meatballs are cooked through and golden brown.

Meanwhile, in a bowl, combine the zucchini slices, grated cheese, breadcrumbs, olive oil, salt and pepper. Mix well to combine the ingredients. Transfer the seasoned courgettes to a baking dish and cook in the preheated oven for about 15-20 minutes, or until the courgettes are tender and golden. Serve the baked beef meatballs with grated courgettes as a side dish. Enjoy your meal!

BAKED COD WITH SAUCE TOMATO AND ARUGULA SALAD

Preparation time: 15 minutes

Cooking times: 20-25 minutes

Ingredients:

Serves 4 people

4 cod fillets

2 cups tomato sauce

2 cloves garlic, minced

2 tablespoons of olive oil

1 teaspoon dried oregano

Salt and pepper to taste.

For the arugula salad:

400 g of fresh arugula

Juice of 1 lemon, 2 tablespoons of olive oil

Salt and pepper to taste.

Preparation:

Preheat the oven to 180°C. In a pan, heat the olive oil and fry the chopped garlic until golden brown. Add the tomato puree, oregano, salt and pepper. Mix well to combine the ingredients. Arrange the cod fillets on a baking tray and pour the tomato sauce over them. Bake in the preheated oven for about 20-25 minutes, or until the cod is cooked through and the sauce is hot and slightly reduced. Meanwhile, in a bowl, mix the arugula, lemon juice, olive oil, salt and pepper to create a salad dressing. Serve the baked cod with the tomato sauce accompanied by the arugula. Enjoy your meal!

STEAMED SALMON WITH SAUTEED ASPARAGUS

Preparation time: 10 minutes

Cooking times: 15-20 minutes

The ingredients:

Serves 4 people

4 salmon fillets

1 bunch of fresh asparagus

Lemon juice

Salt and pepper to taste.

Olive oil

Preparation:

Preheat the oven to 180°C. Place the salmon fillets on sheets of baking paper. Season the salmon with lemon juice, salt and pepper. Close the baking paper to create airtight packages around the salmon. Steam the salmon in the preheated oven for approximately 15-20 minutes, or until cooked through. In the meantime, blanch the asparagus in boiling salted water for a few minutes, then drain. Heat a pan with a drizzle of oil and sauté until crispy. Season the asparagus with salt and pepper. Serve the steamed salmon with the sautéed asparagus.

CHICKEN BREAST STUFFED WITH CHEESE AND SPINACH WITH SAUCEED MUSHROOMS

Preparation time: 15 minutes

Cooking times: 25-30 minutes

Ingredients:

Serves 4 people

4 skinless chicken breasts

cheese (for example ,

mozzarella or provola) , fresh spinach

Salt and pepper to taste, olive oil

Sliced mixed mushrooms

Minced garlic, lemon juice

Chopped fresh parsley

Preparation:

Preheat the oven to 200°C. Prepare the chicken breasts by opening them like a book and stuffing them with slices of cheese and fresh spinach. Close the chicken breasts and secure them with a toothpick. Heat the olive oil in a skillet over medium-high heat and brown the chicken breasts until golden brown. Transfer the chicken breasts to a baking sheet and bake in the oven for about 20 to 25 minutes, or until the chicken is cooked through and the cheese is melted. Meanwhile, in a separate pan, heat the olive oil over medium heat and add the chopped garlic and sliced mushrooms. Fry them until they are tender and golden. Squeeze the lemon juice over the mushrooms and sprinkle them with the chopped parsley. Serve the stuffed chicken breasts with a side dish of sautéed mushrooms.

PAN-FED PRAWNS WITH GARLIC AND PARSLEY SERVED WITH ASPARAGUS

Preparation time: 10 minutes

Cooking times: 5-7 minutes

Ingredients:

Serves 4 people

500 g of fresh prawns , peeled and clean

3-4 cloves of minced garlic

Fresh parsley, chopped

Lemon juice

Salt and pepper to taste.

Olive oil

Preparation:

Heat some olive oil in a skillet over medium-high heat. Add the chopped garlic and sauté for a few seconds. Add the prawns and cook for 2 to 3 minutes per side, until pink and opaque. Season with salt, pepper and lemon juice to taste. Sprinkle with plenty of chopped parsley. Serve the pan-fried prawns with garlic, parsley and a garnish of asparagus.

EGG OMELETE WITH CRISPY BACON AND MIXED SALAD

Preparation time: 10 minutes

Cooking times: 10-12 minutes

Ingredients:

Serves 4 people

6 eggs

Crispy bacon, diced

Grated cheese (optional)

Salt and pepper to taste ., Olive oil

Mixed salad (such as lettuce ,

rocket, radicchio)

Salad dressing (as

balsamic vinegar or olive oil)

Preparation:

Heat some olive oil in a non-stick pan over medium heat. Add the crispy bacon and cook until golden and crispy. Beat the eggs in a bowl, season with salt and pepper. Pour the beaten eggs into the pan with the crispy bacon. Cook the omelette for 5-6 minutes or until lightly browned on the bottom. Using a plate, flip the omelette and cook for another 5-6 minutes. Cut the omelette into wedges and serve hot with the mixed salad dressed to taste.

SIDE DISH RECIPES

AVOCADO AND CUCUMBER SALAD

Preparation time: 10 minutes

Cooking time: 0 minutes

Doses for: 4 people

Ingredients:

2 ripe avocados

2 medium cucumbers

1/2 red onion, finely chopped (optional)

1/4 cup chopped fresh cilantro

2 tablespoons lime juice

1 tablespoon olive oil

Salt and pepper to taste

Preparation

Wash and dry the cucumbers. Cut them in half lengthwise and then into thin slices. Peel and cut the avocados in half. Remove the stone and cut them into cubes. In a large bowl, combine cucumbers, avocado, red onion (if using), cilantro, lime juice, olive oil, salt and pepper. Stir gently to combine. Serve immediately and enjoy the freshness of this salad!

BAKED ASPARAGUS WITH PARMESAN

Preparation time: 15 minutes

Cooking time: 20 minutes

Doses for: 4 people

Ingredients:

1 bunch of fresh asparagus

2 tablespoons of olive oil

Salt and pepper to taste

4 tablespoons grated parmesan

Preparation

Preheat the oven to 200°C. Wash and dry the asparagus. Cut off the woody ends of the stems. Arrange the asparagus on a baking tray. Drizzle with olive oil, salt and pepper. Sprinkle with grated parmesan. Bake for 20 minutes, or until the asparagus is tender and golden. Serve immediately as a side dish or tasty appetizer.

MUSHROOMS STUFFED WITH CHEESE

Preparation time: 20 minutes

Cooking time: 25 minutes

Doses for: 4 people

Ingredients:

20 medium button mushrooms

1 clove garlic, minced

2 tablespoons butter

1/4 cup breadcrumbs

1/4 cup grated cheese

(parmesan, pecorino, gruyere, choice)

2 tablespoons chopped fresh parsley

Salt and pepper to taste

Preparation

Preheat the oven to 180°C. Clean the mushrooms with a damp cloth. Gently peel off the stems, leaving the caps intact. In a pan, heat the butter over medium heat. Saute the minced garlic for about 30 seconds, until fragrant. Add the chopped mushroom stems and cook for 2-3 minutes, or until tender. Remove from the heat and add the breadcrumbs, grated cheese, parsley, salt and pepper. Mix well. Fill the mushroom caps with the prepared mixture. Arrange the stuffed mushrooms on a baking tray lined with baking paper. Bake for 20-25 minutes, or until the mushrooms are golden brown and the filling is hot. Serve hot as a tasty side dish.

BROCCOLI SAUTÉED IN GARLIC BUTTER

Preparation time: 10 minutes

Cooking time: 10 minutes

Doses for: 4 people

Ingredients:

2 medium broccoli

3 tablespoons butter

1 clove garlic, minced

1 cup of water

Salt and pepper to taste

Preparation

Wash the broccoli and cut it into florets. In a pan, heat the butter over medium heat. Saute the minced garlic for about 30 seconds, until fragrant. Add the broccoli florets and cook for 2-3 minutes, stirring frequently. Pour in the water and cook over a covered heat for 5-7 minutes, or until the broccoli is tender but still crunchy . Salt and pepper to taste. Serve immediately as a light and tasty side dish.

GRILLED COURGETTES WITH AROMATIC HERBS

Preparation time: 15 minutes

Cooking time: 10 minutes

Doses for: 4 people

Ingredients:

4 medium courgettes

2 tablespoons of olive oil

1 clove garlic, minced

1/4 cup chopped fresh parsley

1 tablespoon chopped fresh basil

1/2 teaspoon dried thyme

Salt and pepper to taste

Preparation

Wash the courgettes and cut them into longitudinal slices about 1 cm thick. In a large bowl, drizzle the zucchini with olive oil. Add the minced garlic, parsley, basil, thyme, salt and pepper. Mix well to blend the flavors. Heat a grill or nonstick skillet over medium-high heat. Grill the courgettes for 2-3 minutes per side, or until golden brown and lightly marked. Serve immediately as a tasty side dish.

BAKED CAULIFLOWER WITH ALMOND BREADCRUMBS

Preparation time: 20 minutes

Cooking time: 30 minutes

Doses for: 4 people

Ingredients:

1 medium cauliflower

2 tablespoons of olive oil

1/4 cup almond breadcrumbs

2 tablespoons grated parmesan

1/4 cup chopped fresh parsley

Salt and pepper to taste

Preparation

Preheat the oven to 200°C. Wash the cauliflower and cut it into florets. In a large bowl, drizzle the cauliflower florets with olive oil. In a separate dish, mix the almond breadcrumbs, grated parmesan, parsley, salt and pepper. Sprinkle the cauliflower florets with the almond breadcrumb mixture, making sure they are well covered. Place the cauliflower on a baking tray lined with baking paper. Bake for 20-30 minutes, or until cauliflower is golden and crisp. Serve hot as a tasty side dish.

CHINESE CABBAGE AND PEPPER SALAD

Preparation time: 15 minutes

Cooking time: 0 minutes

Doses for: 4 people

Ingredients:

1/2 bok choy, thinly sliced

1 red pepper, cut into strips

1 yellow pepper, cut into strips

1/4 cup red onion

finely chopped (optional)

2 tablespoons of olive oil

2 tablespoons lemon juice

1 tablespoon of apple cider vinegar

1/2 teaspoon mustard seeds

Salt and pepper to taste

Preparation

In a large bowl, combine the sliced bok choy, shredded peppers, and chopped red onion (if using). In a small bowl, whisk together the olive oil, lemon juice, apple cider vinegar, mustard seeds, salt, and pepper. Pour the dressing over the salad and mix well to combine. Serve immediately as a fresh and light side dish.

GRILLED AUBERGINES WITH TOMATO SAUCE

Preparation time: 20 minutes

Cooking time: 30 minutes

Doses for: 4 people

Ingredients:

2 medium aubergines

2 tablespoons of olive oil

Salt and pepper to taste

For the tomato sauce:

400 g of peeled and pureed tomatoes

1 clove garlic, minced

1/4 red onion, finely chopped

1 tablespoon chopped fresh basil

1 tablespoon olive oil

Salt and pepper to taste

Preparation

Wash the aubergines and cut them into slices about 1 cm thick. Brush the aubergine slices with olive oil, salt and pepper. Heat a grill or nonstick skillet over medium-high heat. Grill the aubergines for 2-3 minutes per side, or until golden brown and slightly charred. While the aubergines are cooking, prepare the tomato sauce. In a pan, heat the olive oil over medium heat. Sauté the minced garlic and finely chopped onion for about 30 seconds, until fragrant . Add the peeled and pureed tomatoes, the chopped basil, salt and pepper. Cook over low heat for 15-20 minutes, stirring occasionally, until the sauce has thickened. Once the aubergines are grilled, arrange them on a serving platter. Pour the hot tomato sauce over the aubergines. Serve hot as a delicious side dish.

SAUTÉED SPINACH WITH PINE NUTS AND RAISINS

Preparation time: 10 minutes

Cooking time: 10 minutes

Doses for: 4 people

Ingredients:

500 g of fresh spinach

2 tablespoons of olive oil

2 cloves garlic, minced

50 g of pine nuts

50 g of sultanas

Salt and pepper to taste

Preparation

Wash the spinach carefully and drain it well. In a pan, heat the olive oil over medium heat. Sauté the minced garlic for 30 seconds, until fragrant. Add the pine nuts and cook for 1-2 minutes, stirring constantly, until golden. Add the sultanas and cook for another minute. Add the spinach to the pan and cook for 3-4 minutes, stirring frequently, until wilted. Salt and pepper to taste. Serve the sautéed spinach with pine nuts and raisins immediately as a side dish.

ARUGULA SALAD WITH AVOCADO AND PUMPKIN SEEDS

Preparation time: 15 minutes

Cooking time: 0 minutes

Doses for: 4 people

Ingredients:

200 g of Arugula

1 ripe avocado, cut into cubes

50 g of pumpkin seeds

1/4 cup crumbled feta cheese

2 tablespoons of olive oil

1 tablespoon lemon juice

Salt and pepper to taste

Preparation

Wash the rocket thoroughly and dry it well. In a large bowl, combine the arugula, diced avocado, pumpkin seeds and crumbled feta cheese. In a small bowl, whisk together the olive oil, lemon juice, salt, and pepper. Pour the dressing over the salad and mix well to combine. Serve the arugula salad with avocado and pumpkin seeds immediately as a fresh appetizer or light side dish. Tips: You can also use other types of dried fruit, such as walnuts or almonds, instead of pumpkin seeds. Arugula salad with avocado and pumpkin seeds can also be served as a dressing for pasta or as a filling for sandwiches.

CONCLUSION

"Thank you so much to all our readers for choosing to explore the world of the Atkins Diet 2025 with us . We hope this book has inspired and guided every step of your journey to a healthier, happier life. Your support means a lot for us and we are grateful for the opportunity to share this valuable knowledge with you. Before we conclude, we would like to kindly ask you to share your experience by leaving an honest review about this book. Your opinions are crucial to us and help us improve and continue to offer high-quality, useful resources. Thank you again for your continued support and we wish you all a bright and successful future with your new vision of health and wellness. Thank you!" I hope this book has given you the information and tools you need to start your journey to a healthier, happier life . The Atkins Diet 2025 is an effective and sustainable that can help you lose weight, improve your health and increase your energy. Remember that this is just the beginning of your journey. To achieve lasting results, it is important to adopt a healthy lifestyle that includes a balanced diet, regular physical activity and stress management. I want to thank you for reading my book and for giving me the opportunity to share my passion for health and wellness with you. I wish you all the best on your journey to a healthier and happier life. With love,

[KLARLOCK]

9 798325 817571